The History of Nursing at the M.R.I.

For those members of the Nursing Staff who have worked with me in the wards and clinics at the M.R.I.
Also for Christine.

William Brockbank

The History of Nursing at the M.R.I.

1752–1929

It is a worthy edifying sight
And gives to human kind peculiar grace
To feel kind hands attending day and night
With tender ministry from place to place.
Some prop the head: some from the pallid face
Wipe off the faint cold dews weak nature sheds.
Some reach the healing draught: the whilst, to chase
The fear supreme, around their softened bed.

From the 1779/80 Annual Report,
Thomson's *Castle of Indolence*

Manchester University Press

© 1970 William Brockbank

Published by Manchester University Press
316–324 Oxford Road, Manchester, M13 9NR

SBN 7190 1248 1

Printed in Great Britain at the St. Ann's Press, Park Road, Altrincham

Contents

List of Illustrations

Acknowledgements

My thanks are due to the nurses who have contributed their reminiscences, to Miss W. E. Hector who called my attention to Mrs. Gordon Fenwick's connection with the hospital, to Miss Duff Grant, R.R.C., for some notes about Mrs. Fenwick, to Dr. J. G. Bearn who provided the photograph of his uncle in teddy-bear costume, and to successive secretaries to the hospital whose full and easily legible minutes have made my task so easy. I do not suppose they are in any way responsible for the gaps I have been unable to fill.

I am particularly grateful to my friends Andrew Scott and Harold Blundell. I would have hung my head in shame had the errors they detected been allowed to appear in print. Also to three secretaries who did the typing so expertly, Miss Walton, Mrs. Dickinson and Miss Parkes. The errors were not of their making.

Prologue

Discussions had been going on in coffee houses and elsewhere in Manchester about the founding of a Publick Infirmary. There had been an important meeting in April, 1752, and another on June 23, the proceedings being recorded in *Harrop's Manchester Mercury*:

Manchester, June 23
At a meeting of several gentlemen at the Old Coffee House on Thursday last a subscription was open'd for the support of the intended Infirmary in Manchester. The Rules and Orders for governing it were agreed upon and order'd to be printed and a house (which is already taken) to be furnish'd with all convenient speed and proper notice will be giv'n of the first Weekly Board for the admission of patients.

These first Rules and Orders of the Infirmary were printed in 1752 by 'R. Whitworth, bookseller betwixt the Angel and Bull's Head Inns almost facing the market cross'. They give a clear account of how the hospital was managed.

The government was placed in the hands of certain Trustees. These were persons who had given twenty guineas or upwards at one time and were regarded as Trustees for life, or subscribers of two guineas or upwards annually who were 'Trustees during payment'. The General Board of Trustees was to be held quarterly and was given the power to make or repeal the regulations and to elect and remove the officers. In addition there was a Weekly Board of Trustees consisting of five at least, and meeting every Monday morning at eleven o'clock at the Infirmary, to carry on the routine hospital business. The minutes of these two Boards are preserved in unbroken sequence. The Treasurer, who was regarded as chairman, was elected at the General Board before midsummer and was expected if required to 'give security to such persons as the General Board shall appoint for the due accounting of all such money as he shall receive for the use of the Infirmary'. Visitors were appointed from among the contributors to:

visit the House once every day for the ensuing week . . . to enquire whether the rules concerning officers, servants and patients have been observed; particularly whether the patients have been duly attended by the Physicians, Surgeons, Apothecary, etc., whether prayers have been duly read; whether the patients or servants have been guilty of swearing, drunkenness, any immorality or indecency; whether the provisions are good, and whether they have been carried out of the House or brought in to the patients clandestinely.

It was clearly laid down that no Treasurer, Auditor, Physician or Surgeon was to receive any reward, salary or gratuity from the Infirmary for his service and that 'no patient or person related to the Infirmary should at any time presume on pain of expulsion to give or take from any tradesman, patient, servant, stranger or other person whatsoever any fee, reward or gratuity directly or indirectly for any service done, or to be done, on account of the Infirmary'.

Patients were admitted and discharged every Monday by the Weekly Board between the hours of eleven and one. Candidates for admission had to attend before eleven o'clock. Subscribers of one guinea had the right to recommend one out-patient at a time; subscribers of two guineas, one in-patient or two out-patients at a time; Life Trustees had similar rights and it was a fundamental rule that, except in cases that would not admit of delay, no person should be admitted a patient without a recommendation signed by a subscriber or benefactor. No persons might be admitted who were able 'to subsist themselves or pay for their cure'. Arrangements were made for public prayers to be offered for any patient during his illness, and it was hoped that he would return public thanks in his place of worship upon his recovery.

It was ordered that one Physician and one Surgeon, attending in their turns, must visit the hospital every Monday morning also at eleven o'clock, to examine those recommended as patients and to give their opinions to the Board. They would receive under their care such as were admitted. The Physicians and Surgeons were required to meet every Thursday morning at eleven to visit their in-patients to consult upon difficult cases, to note down the patients fit to be discharged on the Monday following and to prescribe for any out-patients then on their books. They were expected to visit their in-patients at other times as they judged necessary, or on being given notice of any sudden emergency from the Apothecary or Matron. No amputation 'or other great operation' except in cases of urgency was to be performed without a previous consultation of the Physicians and Surgeons.

The Apothecary was responsible for keeping the notes of the patients. He had to visit the wards every morning and supply the Weekly Board with a statement regarding the stock of drugs and medicines. He was not allowed to dispense medicines without the direction of the Physicians and Surgeons, except in cases of necessity when they could not be consulted. He was required to be present when the Physicians and Surgeons attended, and the Matron must always know where he could be found.

The Matron took charge of the household goods and furniture and had to ensure the cleanliness of the chambers, beds, cloths, linen and all things within the hospital. She visited the wards and offices daily to see that the nurses, servants and patients observed the rules and did their duty. She kept a daily account of the provisions and attended to their distribution and in her diet book the number of patients on each diet were listed. All the keys were in her possession and she had to see that the doors were 'always locked at nine in the evening from Michaelmas to Lady Day and at ten in the evening from Lady Day to Michaelmas'.

Nurses were expected to clean their wards by seven in the morning in the summer and by eight in the winter, and serve breakfast an hour later. They and the servants were ordered to obey the Matron 'as their mistress' and to behave with tenderness towards the patients and with civility and respect to strangers. It was essential that they should be free of the burden of children and the care of a family.

Patients were not allowed to leave the hospital without permission or to 'lie out on any account whatsoever on pain of expulsion'. Men were forbidden to go into the women's wards and vice versa without leave of the Matron. Patients of both sexes were forbidden to swear, curse or behave rudely or indecently on pain of expulsion after the first admonition. They might not presume to play cards or dice or any other game or smoke within the walls of the hospital, without leave from the Physicians or Surgeons given through the Matron. Those who were able were expected to nurse the other patients, wash and iron the linen, and clean the wards. They might not loiter about the Infirmary or adjacent streets or beg anywhere in the town, on pain of being discharged for irregularity. Once so discharged they could not be admitted again as a patient on any recommendation whatsoever.

The Founders with their rules drafted soon raised a sufficent fund to enable them to furnish with beds and other necessities their small newly-built house in Garden Street. There is no mention in the minutes of the number of beds but there must have been at least twelve.

Part 1

The Matrons

I

Mrs. Ann Worrall 1752-59
Mrs. Elizabeth Taylor 1759-61
Mrs. Jane Smith 1761-66

The Publick Infirmary in Manchester opened its doors on Monday, July 27, 1752. There was a full meeting of the Board. No in-patients were admitted but there was one out-patient, John Boardman. He was handed over for treatment to Edward Hall, one of the three surgeons present. This happened in a small house in a little street called Garden Street, off Withy Grove, a stone's throw from the present Victoria Station. The first Matron was Mrs. Ann Worrall. She had no nurse, no servant, no porter to help her look after the twelve beds until the hospital had been opened for two and a half months and the beds were kept full. However, early in October she was provided with a servant.

The Matron was not paid a penny apart from her expenses until she had worked almost unaided for five months. She was then paid £3 and given £2 more as a gratuity. The maid was paid half the salary given to the Matron plus a gratuity of £1. Neither received any more cash for six months, when the sum of £9 11s. 8d. was divided between Matron and servant.

In August 1763 the Infirmary was extended into the adjoining house and the number of beds was increased to 24. One nurse, Jane Smith, and one porter were added to the staff and must have been welcome relief to Mrs. Worrall and the servant Ellen Heap. The hospital was so busy that there were at one time 29 patients in the house. The nurse was paid £3 a year but received no money until she had worked for six months. But in February 1754 a kinder policy prevailed. The wages were thereafter paid quarterly in the middle of the quarter.

The houses were far too small for the needs of the growing town so the Board decided to build a hospital in Piccadilly on the site now occupied by the sunken garden. The building faced a pond caused by the digging out of clay used at the time for building purposes. The pond had been used for ducking scolding women, witches and other female malefactors. The hospital was opened in 1755, the church bells ringing in its honour. It remained on the site for 153 years—until December 1908.

No-one can read the Minute Books of the Infirmary without being immensely impressed by the influence the hospital has had on the life of the town. The Infirmary was only eleven years old when its Board decided to build a hospital where persons disordered in their senses could 'expect that humane treatment and judicious advice which they had no encouragement to expect in private mad-houses'. It was built on the Infirmary site. Out of this scheme grew Cheadle Royal.

In 1753 Richard Holt was discharged 'for irregularity on account of his ill treatment of the Matron and disobeying the Physicians and Surgeons, swearing and cursing and other instances of irregularity'. Matrons were changing frequently. Mrs. Worrall stayed for seven years and was then replaced by Mrs. Elizabeth Taylor who held office 'with the usual wages and gratuities' for two years. We are not told why they left. The third Matron was Mrs. Jane Smith. One wonders if she was Mrs. Worrall's first nurse but there is no information on the point, but on June 19, 1766, after she had held office for four and a half years, the following minute appears: 'A ballot being demanded whether Mrs. Jane Smith should be continued as Matron it passed in the negative 32 against 8.' Unfortunately we are not told what she had done wrong. She wasn't the only Matron to be sacked.

2

Mrs. Catherine Fletcher 1766-91
Mrs. Ann Dickenson 1791-98

The fourth Matron stayed longer. She was elected 'for the ensuing year' on July 17, 1766. A year later she was given a gratuity of £6 'for last year's care and services.' Her salary was increased to £20 per annum in 1768. She was given a gratuity of five guineas in 1771 and another in 1774 'for her trouble in providing for the patients in the Lunatic Hospital.' There are some interesting minutes at this period.

1767. Ordered that it be recommended to the Apothecary to call together the patients and other members of this Family and of the Lunatic Hospital on every Sunday evening to read such practical books as shall be appointed by the Chaplains.

1771. Ordered that the following directions be given to the nurses: (1) That every patient has clean sheets upon their first admission. (2) That they have clean sheets at least once in three weeks. (3) That two patients be not suffered to be in the same bed except that there is no spare bed in the house. [This rule should be noted in particular—the practice of putting two patients in one bed was thereby authorized.] (4) That the patients be not suffered to apply poultices without the presence of the nurse. (5) That an assistant be provided for the nurse.

The rules were revised in 1769 and contain tables of diet. A patient on the *low diet* received for breakfast a pint of water gruel or milk pottage. For dinner he was given either a pint of broth and two ounces of roots, or a pint of rice milk or eight ounces of bread pudding. Occasionally he could have two ounces of veal instead of milk pottage, but on Wednesday and Friday he might have as a change an ounce of butter or two ounces of cheese. Throughout the day he was allowed 'bread sufficient without waste' and up to a pint of beer.

The *common diet* was similar to the low diet for breakfast, but for dinner the ration was generous. A patient might have eight

ounces of boiled mutton, beef or veal, and eight ounces of roots, and
a pint of rice milk or twelve ounces of baked pudding. It seems a lot
by modern standards. For supper he was issued with a pint of broth
made to the following recipe: 'For every gallon of broth put in three
pounds of mutton or veal or two pounds of lean beef over and above
the common allowance of meat.' He was given as much bread and
beer as he wanted.

There was also a *milk diet* and a *dry diet*. This last consisted of
an ounce of butter or two ounces of cheese for breakfast and supper.
Dinner was much the same as for the common diet only the ration
was less generous. Bread and sea biscuits were 'issued without
waste'.

The hospital was very busy. By 1777 the Matron was receiving
£25 a year but she was still very short of staff. In 1785 she was
informed that the wages of her nurses had been increased by two
guineas a year. But they were forbidden to take threepence from
in-patients on their admission or any other presents whatever. In
1788 she was provided with more nurses 'so that the legs and arms
of every patient could be washed with soap and water after admission, and that such washing be often repeated unless ordered to the
contrary'.

Early in 1788 Mr. Howard, the prison reformer, who was also
interested in hospitals, visited the Infirmary. He seems to have been
critical about its internal state with the result that the Board ordered
an enquiry into the ventilation and general cleanliness of the wards.
The report was considered and improvements were at once insti-
gated. Windows were altered and enlarged to admit more air.
Proper openings for the admission of air were made between the
wards and galleries. Instructions were given that the floors of all
wards should be cleaned more often with soap and warm water, that
the walls should be whitewashed and the doors and woodwork
covered with turpentine varnish annually, or more often if necessary.

The Matron received another gratuity of £5 in 1788 for her
particular attention in her office as Matron. Three years later she
gave notice of her resignation as from June 24. She was 'unanimously
thanked for her long and faithful service' and was presented with a
piece of plate valued at five guineas.

In 1791 it was ordered that the Matron must take care that every
in-patient had clean sheets when admitted and every fourteen days
during their continuance in the Infirmary and oftener if there be
occasion.

She must take care that the Nurses scour their respective Wards with soap and warm water every Friday before eight o'clock in the morning from the first day of March to the first of October and before nine o'clock from the first of October to the first of March and that they mop in their respective Wards once in every week on an intermediate day before the same hours and keep them constantly clean by sweeping – but that the use of sand be totally abolished.

The Matron must also take care that the Nurses scald the chamber pots every morning and scour them every Tuesday and Friday and that they be kept out of the Wards during the day time, except in cases of necessity.

The Nurses must be particularly attentive to carry as soon as possible all empty phials, gallipots, etc., into the shop and that they do not on any account neglect to administer punctually the medicines as prescribed by the Physicians or Surgeons.

The Nurses must obey the orders of the Physicians, Surgeons, Apothecary and Matron. They must not neglect, insult or quarrel with any patient on any pretext whatever, but if any patients do not observe the Rules hung up in each Ward or otherwise misbehave the Nurses must immediately complain to the Apothecary or Matron, and if the fault be not properly attended to by them the Nurses must inform the House Visitors or Weekly Board of the case.

In addition to the present Nurses a man and a woman were to be appointed, the former of whom should superintend the Men's Wards, and the latter those of the Women, see that the medicines be duly administered in their respective departments and all patients after operations should be attended, take care to provide proper dressings and bandages with which they should be ready to wait on the Surgeons in their particular Wards at the usual hour of dressing and at all times to have a proper supply of the same in cases of emergency. The man must provide dressings and bandages in the Surgery every morning by nine o'clock and perform such other services as the Surgeons shall direct, and that both the man and the woman will be subjected to the Rules made for the government of the Nurses, and the Nurses shall on all occasions relative to their official employments, be responsible to them as they themselves shall be to the House Surgeon and Matron.

The Secretary shall send letters every Friday to seven subscribers in rotation residing in Manchester or Salford, requesting their attendance on the Monday following at the Weekly Board, there to take upon themselves the office of House Visitor.

Mrs. Ann Dickenson was appointed Matron on June 23, 1791. On the same day it was:

Ordered that the thanks of this Board be given to the President, Treasurers and all other officers; also to all the Physicians and Surgeons,

Clergy, Apothecary, Physicians' Clerk, for the very extraordinary pains and meritorious services for the welfare of those extensive charities in their several stations during the last year.

Ordered that the following Rules shall be observed by the Matron and that the same be hung up in her room, viz.,

The Trustees of the Charity require, that you carefully superintend the management of this Infirmary in every particular; and see, that it is conducted with the greatest possible regularity, cleanliness and economy.

That you shall visit all the Wards at least every morning and evening, at which time you shall enquire of the patients whether they have their medicines regularly given them, and whether they are properly attended, and well used by the Nurses. You shall also enquire into the conduct of the patients.

That you shall be careful that each patient has the diet prescribed, that you superintend the cook in preparing it and take care that it is served at a regular stated hour and see that none is wasted, and that neither liquors nor provisions are brought to patients but such as the House provides.

That you treat the patients with good nature and civility, and that you never suffer any degree of cruelty, violence or neglect in the servants towards them to pass uncorrected.

That you pay a strict and unremitted attention to the printed Rules and Orders of this charity and as far as your department extends, see them duly executed.

That you employ no patient in the work of the House without first obtaining leave from his or her Physician or Surgeon.

That in case of improper behaviour from the patients or servants you complain to the Weekly Board.

That you consider yourself in all other cases, as absolutely responsible for the conduct of every servant under your direction.

That no provisions or stores of any kind be purchased without first obtaining your order. That you see there is the quantity charged, and that the quality be good. That you keep the keys of them and that you deliver only such a certain quantity at a time as shall enable you to know that it is consumed by the Charity.

That you never suffer any person to have access to the above provisions or stores without your being present, in order that none may be purloined.

That you lock the gates yourself every evening, which divide the Men's from the Women's Ward.

That you attend the prayers in the Chapel every day, and see that such patients as are able, do the same.

Mrs. Dickenson's salary was increased in 1792 to £30 per annum and she was subjected to further directions:

March 22, 1792
Ordered that the Matron shall be answerable to the Trustees for all linen, china, bed clothes, kitchen furniture, household furniture, provisions and all other articles which are or shall be kept or used in this Infirmary or are or shall be brought into this Infirmary to be kept or used and which shall not be under the Apothecary's care. And that in consideration thereof she shall receive the sum of two guineas annually as an addition to her present salary.

September 30, 1793
Ordered that the Matron acknowledges the receipt of every article brought into the House by signing the initials of her name thereto in its respective account for the satisfaction of the Board.

December 24, 1795
The Matron must devote her whole attention to the business of the House. She shall not make any engagements that may interfere with the interests of the Charity nor absent herself from the House without leaving it in the charge of the Apothecary, it being indispensably necessary that one of them shall always be upon the Premises.

That no other person than the Matron be in possession of any key to any door of the Infirmary or Dispensary except the Porter, who alone shall have possession of that adjoining to his room and that if contrary to this injunction any person within the House shall obtain possession of such keys the Matron lies ordered to give the most early information thereof to the Board.

Mrs. Dickenson resigned on March 22, 1798 'in consequence of her marriage'. The Board advertised for a successor in the following terms:

WANTED
A person to succeed to the office of Matron to these Charities in consequence of the marriage and resignation of Mrs. Dickenson. As the most strict inquiry will be made into the Character and Abilities of the Candidates it will be needless for any persons to apply who have not such requisites as will entitle them to so important a situation.

Possibly the inquiry wasn't strict enough.

3

Mrs. Alice Willoughby 1798-1808

The sixth Matron was an unfortunate choice. There was a contest between Mrs. Willoughby and Mrs. Charlotte Barbor. Upon the vote being taken and collected by ballot, Mrs. Willoughby was declared elected by 86 votes to 52. At first things went well. She was given a gratuity of ten guineas in 1801 on account of her active exertions in the discharge of her duty, especially as the House had been remarkably crowded and many nurses and servants were sick and unable to attend their work. She had other gratuities of ten guineas in 1802, 1804 and 1805 'for constant and faithful discharge of her duties', 1806 and 1807. She was also given permission to add another maid servant to the House in 1806.

But retribution was near for early in 1808 tongues started to wag and Mr. Fox, the house surgeon, brought certain matters to the notice of the Board which caused the appointment of a Committee to inquire into the conduct of the Matron. The report was as follows:

It appears to your Committee that the suspicions which have been entertained to the prejudice of the Matron's character may be comprised under the following heads:

1st. That she has been in the habit of sending a variety of articles from the Infirmary to her daughter (Mrs. Gibson's) house, consisting of milk, butter, fish, ducks, butcher's meat, etc., which caused suspicion to be entertained by the servants that the Charity was defrauded; as it did not appear that such articles were in any way accounted for by the Matron, and in particular the Porter knew of two loads of flour which had been sent there, and which were found to have been paid by the Infirmary as Mr. Heywood's receipt.

2dly. That she received wages for more servants than were employed in her department by the Charity, viz., ten guineas a year for an extra nurse; eight guineas for a dispensary maid and nine guineas a year for two others, who only received from her eight guineas each.

3dly. That on the examination of some bill lately come in for payment from Messrs. Ollivants, Marsdens and Freers, a variety of expensive articles are charged, highly improper in a Charity of this nature, some of which likewise do not appear in the House.

4thly. That articles have been bought and entered under false heads, in particular nine hams from Heywoods which are called in his account 'cheese' and were considered as such in the Infirmary books.

5thly. That heavy boxes have been sent from the Infirmary suspected to contain the property of the Charity, and that when she has gone from home she has taken along with her, beef, tongues, flour, sugar, butter and cheese.

6thly. That there has been an unnecessary consumption of Port wine, a certain quantity of which has been confided to her, but which does not appear to have been consumed in the channels for which it was allowed.

The foregoing points being either substantiated by evidence or admitted by Mrs. Willoughby, she was desired to explain her conduct to the Committee; when she commenced by the most solemn assurances of her innocence; and of having never abused the confidence placed in her, but at the same time commenting that she had acted upon a system recommended by her predecessor, of permitting articles to be entered under false titles, for fear the Officers of the Charity should notice what might appear extravagant or unnecessary. When the milk and butter which were proved to have been regularly sold to her daughter was mentioned, she produced the sum of £45. 6s. which she said arose from that and other sources, of which 17 guineas were collected prior to Midsummer last and £27. 9s. since that time. Upon the apparent inconsistency of this statement being urged, she explained it by saying that all the money which she from time to time received, she regularly put into a drawer, and when anything was wanted in the house which she thought would be disapproved by the Board she purchased it from this fund; but without being able to state any particulars of the amount of her receipts or expenditure in this department, which she professed to keep entirely distinct from the regular house book that is kept with the Secretary.

That during the late Secretary's life she was in the constant habit of paying him every two or three months the balance of this private drawer for some years past; but no entries of this nature appear in his books to her credit.

Mr. Eadon, the present Secretary, recollects that she one day spoke to him concerning some account she had to settle with him, but cannot say of what nature—this she refers to as an intended payment of a balance of her private account, a confirmation of her former settlement with Steadman.

That respecting the money paid her on account of wages, she says that the number of servants differs continually, and that although there may not be an extra nurse and dispensary maid constantly engaged, that there frequently are such servants as well as other assistants to whom she pays weekly wages, and that the remainder has been expended in tea for them. This, however, the servants positively deny, saying they have had none but the remains from the Parlour (which was paid for under a distinct head) until since these enquiries have been made or within about ten days past.

That respecting the furniture she says when she came to the Infirmary, nine or ten years ago on her appointment as Matron, she brought all her stock of every description along with her and that her recent purchases have been made in lieu of it. She never had an Inventory of such furniture as she brought, but she states it to have been considerable in quantity and comprising bedding, glasses and other articles of value.

That nine hams were really bought from Heywoods, entered under the head of cheeses, by her orders, for the reason before stated, and that the quantity consumed would appear considerable to the Board as the Gentlemen frequently required lunches in the fore-noon.

That with regard to fish, ducks, butchers' meat, etc., sent to her daughter's house, the Committee might be assured that everything of that nature was purchased with Mrs. Gibson's money and only came accidentally to the Infirmary where the accommodation for keeping butchers' meat or feeding ducks for a few days was much greater than at her own house, and that to use her own words, the Charity had never been injured to the value of a sprig of parsley, and that she frequently received fish as presents from a distance which she divided with Mrs. Gibson.

In explanation of the two loads of flour, she says that the Porter was directed to order them for Mrs. Gibson and that Heywood must charge them to her, which the Porter positively denies, saying he bought them as usual for the Infirmary, where they were delivered and afterwards sent by half loads to Mrs. Gibson's house.

In her letter to the Committee she admits that she is debtor for that money, but throws the blame upon the Porter, whose story is consistent whilst hers has varied considerably.

It was both proved and admitted by Mrs. Willoughby that on her going from home, she put up three tongues, a piece of roasted beef, a pillow case filled with flour, butter, loaf sugar and parts of two cheeses. On her being interrogated upon these points, she said she had paid for them into the drawer or purchased them on her own account; but on further enquiry, she defended taking them 'as any other person would' for that where she was going she could not have anything of the kind.

A somewhat similar explanation was given of the four heavy boxes sent from the Infirmary, which she said contained many old clothes and other things not specified, as well as currant loaves and sweet wine for her grandchildren which were sent by her daughter to the Infirmary to be packed there, and from whence the carrier's cart fetched them.

The regular supply of about four bottles weekly of port furnished for the purpose of making sago or for the patients, did not appear to your Committee to have been used for such purposes, as the wine really employed was of another description, and that very little pure port is consumed by the patients in sago and gruels.

The bottles which appear to have been frequently sent to Mrs. Gibson's under the idea of being lent, are now said to be taken in exchange for a quantity she brought along with her on coming to the Infirmary.

Without adverting to other matters, which scarcely admit of proof, your Committee are unanimously of opinion that her conduct has been highly irregular in the circumstances of the false entries and the appropriation of money received as servant wages and applied to other purposes, and it remains for the Board to determine how far her general good character and the excuses she has made will or ought to militate in her favour. Whether fraud has been committed in the articles of the unaccounted purse depends entirely upon the Matron's integrity, whose character has hitherto been irreproachable and whose conduct has gained her the confidence of the Trustees at large as well as the Officers of the Charity.

It ought to be mentioned that whatever has been sent from the Infirmary has gone in the face of day and been carried by the servants of the Charity, which does not wear the aspect of conscious guilt; but the Committee feels concerned in stating that facts have come out in the course of these inquiries that considerably diminish the credit which would always be due to the Matron's assertions; but which have very materially differed in the course of three examinations, perhaps all equally remote from the real truth.

Your Committee is of opinion that the Charity is much indebted to Mr. Fox for the perseverance he has shown in the pursuit of this business, to which he was led by some hints communicated by his predecessor who was not able to substantiate any facts sufficiently to ground an accusation upon. This conduct it is hoped will be imitated by every other person employed by the Infirmary, for although it may frequently be a thankless office, it is a duty which everyone of able mind will feel when peculation is suspected, or a noble institution perverted to private advantage. He that connives at what he considers wrong is involved in the guilt and Mr. Fox has, upon this occasion, set an excellent example for which he invites the esteem of every real friend of the Charity.

The Committee cannot conclude without earnestly recommending to the Board that an Order shall be made that any tradesman being found guilty of conniving with the servants of the Charity in making false entries, or entering goods under wrong titles, shall never again be employed by this Institution.

The decision rested with a special Board and at that meeting Mrs. Willoughby produced a long answer in writing to all the criticisms that had been raised. She blamed the porter for having 'malicious design to found a charge' against her. She told the Board that 'as the years increase all the faculties of the mind are greatly impaired and generally sooner in those who have been afflicted with sickness'. Finally she admitted that 'some irregularities had occurred which cannot be justified'.

The Board decided that, 'Mrs. Willoughby, the present Matron, be dismissed from her office in the Infirmary, she having appeared to be unworthy of future confidence.' Mr. Fox, the house surgeon, was publicly thanked for bringing forward the charges against her and hope was expressed that no person in any official situation in the hospital will overlook or conceal anything in the conduct of servants of the Charity injurious to its interests.

Tradesmen and shopkeepers were warned that false entries concealing the real expenses of the Charity would result in the loss of their trade. Finally it was said that great care must be taken in the appointment of a new Matron.

4

Mrs. Charlotte Barbor 1808-15
Mrs. Sarah Loftus 1815-30
Miss Martha Leigh 1830-46

Mrs. Charlotte Barbor was appointed Matron on March 24, 1808, 'in place of Mrs. Willoughby lately dismissed'. It is hardly surprising to find that she was confronted with a new set of 'Rules for the Matron'.

1st. That she shall devote her whole attention to the business of the House, and that she shall not make any engagements that may interfere with the interests of the Charity, nor absent herself from the House without leaving it in charge of the Apothecary. It being indispensably necessary that one of them shall be always upon the premises.

2nd. That she shall take care of the household goods and furniture according to the inventory given her and be ready to give a notice thereof when required.

3rd. That she shall examine, weigh, and measure all the provisions and stores that are brought into the house to ascertain their quantity and quality and see that every article is entered in the books kept for that purpose. That she shall never suffer any person to have access to the stores without being herself present.

4th. That she shall visit the wards and offices every day and take care that the chambers, beds, clothes, linen, and all other things in the house be kept clean; that every In-Patient have clean sheets when admitted and that they be changed every fourteen days, or oftener if necessary.

5th. That books be kept with every tradesman employed in which each article shall be entered at the time it is purchased and that nothing shall be sold or disposed of belonging to the Charity without the knowledge of the Board, and that she keep a cash account of her receipts and expenditure to be examined and balanced on the second Monday in each month by the house steward.

6th. That she take care that the nurses scour their respective wards with soap and warm water every Friday before eight in the morning from the 1st of March to the 1st of October, and before nine o'clock from the

1st of October to the 1st March, and that they mop the wards once in every week on an intermediate day before the same hours and keep them constantly clean by sweeping, and that the use of sand be totally abolished in the wards.

7th. That she take care that the nurses scald the chamber pots every morning and scour them every Tuesday and Friday, and that they be removed out of the wards during the day, except in cases of necessity.

8th. That she see that the nurses, servants and patients observe the Rules of the House and do their duty; and that she be empowered to hire women servants and nurses, and to dismiss them for misbehaviour, being accountable only to the Board, when called upon. In case of ill conduct on the part of the patients she will acquaint the Weekly Board or House Visitors.

9th. That she take care that each patient has the diet prescribed regularly served, and that none of it be wasted with her knowledge, and likewise prevent any liquors or provisions being brought to the patients by their friends.

10th. That she shall treat the patients with civility and good nature and never suffer any degree of insolence or neglect in the servants to pass unnoticed.

11th. That whenever the weather will permit she shall order a certain number of the mattresses, blankets and quilts to be exposed to the sun, in rotation, and well aired, and that such patients as are permitted by the Faculty, shall assist the nurses in the performance of this duty.

12th. That she take care of the keys of the House and sees that the doors be always locked at ten in the evening from Michaelmas to Lady Day and at eleven from Lady Day to Michaelmas, and that no other person be in possession of a key to any door of the Infirmary or Dispensary, except the Porter who alone shall have that of the door adjoining to his room; and that if contrary to this injunction, any person shall obtain possession of such keys, she shall give the most early information to the Board; and that she likewise takes care that the gates which separate the Men's and Women's Wards be locked every evening.

13th. That she make a point of attending prayers in the Chapel every day when divine service is performed and is not prevented by unavoidable business, and sees that such patients as are able do the same.

Mrs. Barbor received a gratuity of ten guineas in 1809. She resigned on January 9, 1815, writing the following letter to the Board:

It is not without a grateful sense of the confidence which I have uniformly experienced from the Trustees as Matron of the Infirmary that I now beg them to accept my resignation of that office. Various circumstances have combined to lead to this determination. I should be sorry however that so excellent an Institution should suffer any inconvenience. I shall therefore continue to fulfil the duties of my situation till a successor can conveniently be appointed and I beg to add that it will afford me heartfelt satisfaction should it be deemed desirable to render any assistance in my power till she becomes acquainted with the business of the House.

The Board accepted her resignation and acknowledged her services in having assiduously attended to the interests of the Charity and in the faithful discharge of her duty. They appointed the eighth Matron, Mrs. Sarah Loftus, on June 22, 1815, and eighteen months later advanced her salary from £30 to £40 per annum. There is a pen-picture of the interior of the wards in a letter dated 1816 from one of the surgeons to the Board.

The imperfect manner in which the wards of the Infirmary are now warmed has probably not escaped your notice. It is self-evident that a small open fire is quite insufficient for the comfortable warming of a large ward and that the crowding up of convalescent patients around it during the day will prevent those who are confined at the lower end from deriving much benefit from it, chilled by cold as they must therefore be in severe weather. The apertures for ventilation are closed and the free circulation of air is in consequence prevented. All of you must likewise occasionally have observed the smoky state of the wards, which from the bad construction of the chimneys in many, it is impractical to remedy.

It was suggested that the Board should give consideration to the heating of the buildings by steam and it was readily agreed to do this. But there were obvious difficulties to be surmounted, and the matter was delayed. It was easier to provide warm baths, one for men, the other for women, suffering from the effects of rheumatism.

The Minute Books are still full of interest. In 1822 a contract was signed for a year's supply of the best meat at 5d. a pound. For coarse meat 'boned and given in' the price was 3d., the meat to be to the satisfaction of the stewards. Milk was supplied at 2s. 4d. per dozen quarts.

In 1824 it was recorded that for some time past a great number of patients could not be admitted into the House in consequence of the crowded state of the wards. The Board therefore decided to obtain plans and estimates for a big extension. Another determining factor was the prevalence of erysipelas in the surgical wards due in part, it was thought, to overcrowding. The estimates amounted to

£7,000, but it was considered that this was far too big a sum to be found from the hospital funds. A special appeal was therefore launched. The scheme chosen necessitated the extension of the original north and south wings, bringing them in line with the main frontage of the two hospitals facing the pond. In addition, the north wing built in 1792 was to be enlarged and this and the main front of the hospital covered with stone. Two porticos were included, one facing the pond and the other Mosley Street. Unfortunately the appeal was not as successful as had been hoped. Though it had brought in £5,600, the Board decided to modify the scheme and start the alterations right away, omitting the cosmetic items but going ahead with vital extensions.

1828. It having been proved that Margaret Bourne, a patient of Dr. Mitchell, had had spiced bread brought into the House and the bread of the House having been brought in and examined and declared by the Medical and other Gentlemen present, good, and more wholesome, the said Margaret Bourne was called in, when she stated she could not eat the bread of the House, and on being asked why she could not, did not give any sufficient reason but behaved improperly to the Board.

Resolved unanimously: That in consequence of the breach of the rules as well as of the improper behaviour of the said Margaret Bourne before the Board she be immediately discharged. (What occurred on this regrettable occasion is not recorded in the Minutes, but the story has come down another way. Margaret Bourne spat on the table.)

The wards were very unhealthy. Wounds became infected and poured pus. Mortality was high; operations were an appalling risk. This applied to hospitals all over the world. The nature of infection and the causes were unknown.

The new buildings were opened early in 1828. There were new wards containing accommodation for 'upwards of sixty additional patients'; three other bedrooms, four nurses' kitchens and eight water closets, a large new washhouse and laundry 'both on the fireproof plan', two extensive kitchens, larder, dairy and storerooms, a large new dining-room, rooms for the resident Apothecary, the physicians' clerks and apprentices; a large accident room and surgery; and other less important structures. The improvements brought more difficulties however. The Matron complained of the great inconvenience to patients in the new wards near the Asylum caused by the drying of clothes of the lunatic patients. The pigsties belonging to that hospital also became a nuisance. There were now upward of 180 beds in the hospital and the new beds were filled at once.

In 1830 the Medical Committee suggested to the Board that in its view it was 'desirable to denominate this Institution a Royal Infirmary'. The Board agreed and drew up a statement for presentation to the King through the Earl of Stamford. The King agreed and the same year the Hospital became known as 'The Manchester Royal Infirmary, Dispensary and Lunatic Hospital'.

We hear something of one of the nurses in 1830: 'In consideration of the faithful services of Ann Leech who has been a nurse in this Institution for upwards of thirteen years and the inability of her friends to pay the expenses of her funeral, it was ordered that the expenses should be paid by the Institution.' In the same year there was a note of a practice that was to continue regularly in the future: 'Ordered that the Matron's room be reserved on the day of the election of Surgeons for the Ladies who are Trustees.' Elections to the Honorary Medical Staff were made at special meetings of the Trustees. Much canvassing took place, often at considerable expense to the applicants. In March 1830 the Matron was given a gratuity of ten guineas but it was too late to prevent her resignation which she asked permission to give the following month 'with every feeling of respect'.

The Board advertised for a Matron. She must have attained thirty years of age and possess a thorough knowledge of housekeeping. She was required to devote her whole attention to the business of the House and must not make any engagements which may interfere with the interests of the Charity. Applicants having families will not be deemed equally eligible with those who have none. The salary was forty guineas per annum, with board and suitable accommodation in the House. It should be noted that no experience of nursing was required.

There were four applicants. All were interviewed and their testimonials were read. Two candidates seemed particularly well qualified and a ballot between them ensued. Miss Martha Leigh got 195 votes and Miss Hatton 182. Miss Leigh was declared elected and directed to enter on the duties of her office on June 24 next. She received gratuities of ten guineas almost every year and was given leave of absence for two or three weeks annually, her duties being carried out by a Mrs. Armstrong. She also had some sick leave. In 1832 it was considered that 'a change of air was necessary for the more speedy and perfect restoration of her health'. Four years later she had a bilious fever and was given leave of absence to allow her to go to her sister's home near Liverpool.

The Matron had a brush with the Apprentices in 1834:

May 19, 1834
To the Chairman of the Weekly Board
Sir,

We the undersigned apprentices of the Institution beg leave most respectfully to call the attention of the Board to institute an enquiry concerning our diet in general.

We are induced to impress this subject more fully upon your consideration finding that the representation we made to you some time ago on the same subject has not produced the slightest alteration and has not been received with the proper attention it ought to have done by the Matron.

Hoping that this appeal will not pass unnoticed we beg leave, Sir, respectfully to subscribe ourselves

Your obedient humble servants,

Charles Snape,
John Henry Brown,
Thomas Richardson,
John Broadhurst,
Wm. Cardwell Beattie,
Edward Tomlinson.

On May 26, 1834, following an enquiry into the above complaint it was resolved unanimously that: 'It is very much regretted that a representation so unfounded should have been addressed to the Board.'

She had trouble with the House Surgeon about the same time: 'The Board having heard the statements of Miss Leigh and Mr. Beever on the subject of his ordering breakfast and tea at irregular hours resolved unanimously that Mr. Beever be informed that the rules respecting the attendance at meals are to be enforced and that he is expected to conform to them.' Times do not change!

It is curious that throughout all these years there is no indication of the number of operations that were taking place. However, in 1833 the Board requested the house-surgeons to produce a statement of the number of operations performed by each surgeon during the last two years. The statement is most interesting. In that period Mr. John Thorp had operated on five occasions only, Mr. Ransome on fifteen, Mr. Ainsworth on twelve, Mr. Robert Thorpe on fifteen, Mr. Wilson on twenty-seven and Mr. Turner on twenty. The 110 operations were described as follows: Amputation of the leg, 40; Amputation of the arm, 22; Hernia, 8; Tumours, 8; Lithotomy, 7;

Contracture after burns, 6; Cataract, 9; Trepan, 3; Aneurysm, 2; Tracheotomy, 2; Hare-lip, 1; Various, 2. It should be remembered that in those days anaesthetics were unknown.

The new accommodation for in-patients in the main hospital soon proved inadequate. It was therefore decided to provide 'twenty new beds with proper bedding' in a room belonging to the Asylum. This should have brought the number of available beds to somewhere in the region of 200, but does not seem to have done so.

The year 1836 and those that followed brought the usual collection of major and minor worries to the notice of the Board. It was recognized that the building was quite inadequate for dealing with the daily increasing number of applicants, but for the time being money was not available for large extensions. The Waterworks Company had to be requested to throw more water into the pond so as to cover the weeds that had grown to the surface. It does not sound a choice place in which to drown, but a woman did drown there. So it became necessary to erect railings between the garden and the pond. The amount of gas consumed by the clock and the lamps outside the hospital was another source of worry. It was pointed out that these were public amenities and had nothing to do with the working of the hospital. In the end the gas company decided to subscribe thirty guineas annually to the hospital funds and this offer was gratefully accepted.

Much more serious was the fact that the surgical wards were extremely overcrowded, and there was an 'exceedingly objectionable practice of putting two patients into one bed'. The problem of the surgical wards was a nightmare to the Board and the Medical Committee. No one at that time knew the cause of infection, nor was it realised that such inflammatory troubles as erysipelas could be carried from patient to patient on apparently clean hands and dressings. Antisepsis and asepsis were unknown and were to remain unknown until Joseph Lister published his famous paper thirty years later. In an effort to improve these wards the Medical Committee advised that the floors should be dry-rubbed instead of washed. The Matron disapproved and the Board agreed to the experiment rather unwillingly. After several months the Medical Committee reported happily but perhaps unwisely that its prediction had proved correct. The wards were healthier and there had not been one case of erysipelas that had originated in the Hospital. The Board therefore re-drafted the rules for the Matron and nurses so as to legalize the new method.

c

The number of operations was beginning to increase. In a two-year period (1838–1840) there had been 143 with a mortality of thirty-six (25 per cent). It was decided to publish the return of operations annually, but on this particular occasion the mortality figures were not given.

To combat the overcrowding, fourteen extra beds were added in 1841, making a total of 192 beds, 67 medical and 125 surgical. These figures do not agree with those previously given, for the number should have been about 214. Possibly this discrepancy is accounted for by the double beds which the Board had recently decided should hold one patient only.

Ventilation in the wards was still unsatisfactory, particularly in the newer blocks. It was suggested that this could be improved if movable panels were placed in the doors. This had little or no effect, so in 1844 the opinion of an architect was obtained. He found that the 'vitiated air' from the kitchens, the lower wards and the offices ascended by the spacious galleries and staircases to the upper parts of the building, where it made its way into the different apartments, the atmosphere of which was already overloaded with impurities. In one part of the building over the dispensary, where the servants slept, he found he had difficulty in breathing, because this was the highest part of the inside of the buildings and the impure air ascended thither with no means of escape. In those days, of course, servants hardly dared to breathe.

The principal means of ventilation was by the doors and windows, which subjected the wards to local draughts and the patients to all the evil consequences arising therefrom. Various methods were proposed to improve the trouble. Meanwhile, as the house was particularly unhealthy, the Board respectfully asked the Medical Committee to make a weekly statement on the health of the patients in the wards. At this period, 1843–44, the mortality rate was high (12 per cent, compared with 5 per cent in 1947–48). At once it became apparent that things very unsatisfactory in the surgical wards.

Eight cases with in-patient recommendations could not be admitted for want of room.

The house was as usual crowded. Eight double beds were in use.

Twelve double beds were in use.

The house-surgeon reported the house was crowded and unhealthy.

The house-surgeon reported the house was being white-washed.

The house-surgeon reported that the house was crowded and un-healthy – four double beds were in use. The order of the Board has been strictly adhered to in reserving twelve beds for accidents instead of three, still the house remains so crowded that it has been impossible to prevent the use of double beds though some accidents of severe nature have been refused admission.

Erysipelas again prevails and the patients are all more or less suffering from the very unhealthy state of the surgical wards.

At other times things were better: 'The house-surgeon reported that the house was crowded but very healthy: four double beds.' But more often than not it was an unhealthy report. There was only one thing to be done. The Hospital must be extended on a big scale and in 1845 it was decided to proceed with the job.

Meanwhile other things of importance were happening. In 1838 it was 'resolved that the Matron be informed that the cook's wages are for the future to be fifteen guineas per annum without the remuneration hitherto derived from the sale of dripping and other perquisites whatever'.

In the same year she ran into trouble with the Medical Committee, who asked that the wards should be dry-rubbed instead of washed, but Miss Leigh said there were obstacles to this being carried out. They asked what these were, and when told they considered them 'frivolous and unimportant'. They said dry rubbing appeared to be absolutely necessary as a means of preventing the great mortality from infection in the hospital. The Board instructed her to attend to the more efficient performance of the dry cleaning. In 1840 the Medical Committee complained that the wards were still being washed and not dry rubbed and that several cases of erysipelas had followed – two of them fatal. The Board instructed her to attend to the more efficient performance of the dry cleaning. Miss Leigh stated that she thought the spirit of the resolution had been carried with effect but that in future she would take care that both in the spirit and in the letter the directions should be strictly conformed with. No one yet knew anything about bacteria or the nature of infection, but, to the modern mind, dry scrubbing would have raised a bacterial dust. Wet washing would have been much more hygienic.

Miss Leigh applied for an advance in salary in 1840, but only received a gratuity of ten guineas 'in consideration of her long and efficient services in the execution of her duty'. The gratuity was raised to twenty guineas in 1842.

It was decided in 1843 to commission a Corporate Seal at a cost of sixteen pounds. This showed the Good Samaritan in the act of relieving the wounded traveller. Above the picture was the motto *Vade et tu fac similiter.*

The problem of the surgical wards was still a nightmare to the Board and to the Medical Committee. Nobody realised that bacteria could be carried from patient to patient on apparently clean hands and dressings. The number of operations was beginning to increase. It reached seventy in a year for the six surgeons. One operation a month for each of them, mortality 25 per cent.

Earlier in 1846 the members of the Medical Committee expressed the opinion that the nurses of the hospital were for the most part inefficient. Accordingly the Board decided that two upper nurses or sisters should be appointed, one for the medical and one for the surgical department, at a salary that should not exceed twenty-five pounds per annum. The Medical Committee did not like this idea and suggested that there should be no alteration of the duties of the present nurses, there being one upper nurse for each sex whose duties were well defined and whose work in general had been efficiently discharged. But in the surgical department without any change in the present system it was desirable to secure the services of more efficient nurses. It was therefore suggested that 'no nurse should be engaged without the sanction of the Medical Committee'.

The Board therefore endeavoured to secure superior nurses by increasing their salary to not less than twelve pounds per annum and paying each night nurse not less than two shillings a night.

You may think the Matron is all powerful now, but I wonder if she was not even more so in 1847 when we find the following minute:

Inquiry having been made relative to the consumption of beer, it was unanimously resolved that all luncheons to students be discontinued. That the allowance for the residents' dining room be one pint of beer for each person at dinner and supper. That the male servants be allowed each a pint of beer for dinner and supper. Resolved that a tap be placed under the control of the Matron for supplying beer and a daily account be kept of the same.

The usual gratuity of twenty guineas was paid to Miss Leigh in June 1846. Five months later she resigned. The Board 'lamented' that her letter had not been sent at an earlier date. No explanation is given for this cryptic remark. But the Board thanked her handsomely in the following minute:

The Board, duly sensible of Miss Leigh's unwearied zeal and constant attentions to the welfare of the Charity during the period of sixteen years in which she has held the arduous and truly responsible situation of Matron, present to her a gratuity of thirty guineas in consideration of her long and faithful services. It is directed that a copy of the resolution be transmitted to her by the Secretary.

Miss Leigh acknowledged the resolution saying it was a source of great satisfaction to her that her services had been thought deserving of so handsome a testimonial and so liberal a gratuity.

Up to now it has been impossible to get any idea of the sort of women who became nurses. They are never mentioned in the Minutes and only very occasionally does the Matron appear. But in 1844 Charles Dickens wrote *Martin Chuzzlewit* and therein depicted Mrs. Sairey Gamp and her scarcely less famous colleague, Mrs. Betsy Prig, both immortal portraits. Nurses in the 19th century were a poor class of women. It needed the forceful pen of Dickens to show how degraded they were and the depths to which the ordinary professional nurse had sunk. He was deliberately indulging in propaganda. Twenty-four years later he wrote:

Mrs. Sarah Gamp was a fair representation of the hired attendant on the poor in sickness. The Hospitals of London were, in many respects, noble institutions: in others very defective. I think it is not the least among the instances of this mismanagement, that Mrs. Betsy Prig was a fair specimen of a hospital nurse and that the hospitals . . . should have left it to private humanity and enterprise to enter on an attempt to improve that class of persons – since greatly improved through the agency of good women.

Eleven years later Florence Nightingale found that only sixteen out of the thirty-eight nurses she took out to Scutari were really satisfactory.

5

Miss Margaret Macmillan 1846-50
Mrs. Jessie Harding 1851-55
Miss Maria Owtram 1854-65

Miss Macmillan was elected by ballot on December 3, 1846. New rules were made in 1849, including the following:

> That the nurses for the medical wards be appointed and dismissed by the Resident Medical Officer and Matron conjointly and the nurses for the surgical wards be appointed and dismissed by the Resident Medical Officer, the House Surgeon and Matron conjointly. In the appointment or dismissal of any nurse if the Resident Medical and Surgical Officers and Matron differ in opinion the case shall be referred to the Treasurer and House Stewards for final decision.

Miss Macmillan resigned on December 2, 1850, saying she wished to leave before Christmas.

> The Board had great pleasure in recording the high sense it entertains of the very efficient and economical manner in which she has conducted the important duties of her office and desires to express its sincere wishes for her health and happiness in her new sphere of life also that a copy of the resolution be forwarded to Mrs. Whaley (late Miss Macmillan) by the Secretary.

There is no note in the Minutes that she ever received a gratuity. I can find no record in the minutes of the appointment of her successor Mrs. Jessie Harding, but her name is recorded as Matron in the list of office bearers published in June 1851. Up to now there has been no mention of the sleeping accommodation for the nurses, but in 1853 it is stated that there were rooms in the basement for one sub-matron, five night nurses and fifteen day nurses. By now the Matron was receiving a salary of seventy guineas with board and suitable accommodation in the house. Mrs. Harding resigned on January 29, 1855, without giving any reason. The Weekly Board at once issued an advertisement for a successor:

Each candidate for the post must have attained thirty years of age and had to possess a thorough knowledge of housekeeping [It is odd that a knowledge of nursing was still not included in the advertisement.] She was required to devote her whole morning to the business of the hospital and was not allowed to make any engagements which might interfere with her work.

Although this was at the end of January the Quarterly Board minutes for December 21 (five weeks earlier) record that Miss Maria Owtram was Matron. This was certainly 'jumping the gun' for Miss Owtram succeeded to the post. She does not appear in the minutes until September 1857 when she was given two or three weeks' leave of absence starting on October 2.

Diet tables came under review in 1859. The old tables were not being obeyed and there were many complaints, particularly about potato pie and potato hash. Because of this, patients were given the generous diet or the extra diet which were more expensive. The surprising thing was that 'thick pie crust made with suet could have formed an article of food for invalids for so many years'. The hash was made with warmed-up meat cooked the previous day. No attempt was made to flavour it. No butter was served at tea-time. It seemed wrong to serve patients with gruel at eleven o'clock at night. There was too much sameness in the milk diets. More beer than was necessary or beneficial was allowed to all patients. Most of the patients did not drink beer in their homes.

It was found that changes could be made to the advantage of the patients with pecuniary profit to the Charity. Potato pie was discontinued. Potato hash was made to a special recipe with cold meat, potatoes and bread as an alternative choice. Butter was served at tea-time and treacle was banned from the wards. Milk puddings were more varied. Beef tea was supplied. For the generous diet there was a choice of roast or boiled beef or mutton. Beer could only be ordered specially instead of a pint being supplied to each patient. For breakfast there was now a choice of tea or coffee. It was found that two-thirds preferred coffee.

In 1858 the Medical Wards supplied five times the number of generous diets compared to common diets. After the change the numbers were four common to three generous and a 'very decided falling off of the extra diets (mutton chops and fowl)'. There was in fact a striking difference between the figures of the medical and surgical wards, the surgical wards lagging far behind with a steady increase in the extra diets.

Medical Wards (lbs.)	1858	1859
Common Diet	482	1604
Generous and Extra Diets	2630	1290
Surgical Wards (lbs.)		
Common Diet	4188	4304
Generous and Extra Diets	3221	3221
Consumption of Beer (pts.)		
Medical Wards	1801	750
Surgical Wards	6330	1067

New Diet Tables were drawn up:

Generous Diet
Breakfast: One pint tea or coffee, 6 oz. bread, ¾ oz. butter, or boiled bread and milk or porridge with milk.
Dinner: On four days 6 oz. beef roasted, 4 oz. bread, 8 oz. potatoes. On the three alternate days 6 oz. mutton boiled instead of the beef. This diet was changed in alternate weeks to boiled beef and roast mutton.
Supper: The same as breakfast but no coffee allowed.

Common Diet
Breakfast: As above but one ounce less bread and a quarter ounce less butter.
Dinner: On three days as above (roast beef). On one day one pint of good soup, 2 oz. roast meat and potatoes, 4 oz. bread. On three days potato hash with 4 oz. bread or the option of having cold meat with 8 oz. potatoes and 4 oz. bread.
Supper: As for breakfast but no coffee.

Milk Diet
Breakfast: As for the Common Diet.
Dinner: ½ pint of milk each day with either 12 oz. semolina pudding (2 days), 12 oz. rice pudding (3 days), 12 oz. bread pudding (2 days). At the option of the medical and surgical officers ½ pint beef tea could be substituted for ½ pint milk.
Supper: As for breakfast but no coffee.

Low Diet
Breakfast: One pint tea, 3 oz. bread.
Dinner: One pint gruel, 2 oz. bread.
Supper: Water gruel or tea, 3 oz. bread.

Arrangements were made for the dietary on the wards to be inspected regularly and for a monthly report to be made to the Board.

September 5, 1859
Greater care and attention is needed in sending up from the kitchen suitable meat for making beef tea. In one specimen submitted to the

Committee one pound of fat was removed from 3½ lbs. meat. No fat whatever should be sent to the nurses' kitchen for the purpose of beef tea making.

December 5, 1859
Extras are occasionally ordered on the Medical Wards not comprehended in the diet list such as custard puddings and beef steak puddings. Semolina puddings are given on days when they do not occur in the list, while one patient lately discharged has had no less than 26 mutton chops for breakfast.

January 9, 1860
There has been a steady rise in the article mutton chops since September, the monthy returns being 47, 48, 78, 98, 158.

February 6, 1860
The diet tables in the surgical wards continue to show a steady increase of extras: chops, fowl and fish. There is something radically wrong here. The regulations set forth in the diet tables are not properly adhered to. Either the tables are right or wrong and if wrong the properly constituted authorities should rectify them.

This caused the Treasurer and House Stewards to interview the Matron, Cook and House Surgeon and arrangements were made which, it was confidently hoped, would prevent in future such breaches of the Diet Tables. This had a salutory effect.

June 11, 1860
The fowl and chop diets are all but doubled. This may be accounted for by there being three diabetic cases, reputed incurable.

December 17, 1860
Fowls cost 1s. 6d. and make four dinners.

Patients were rarely mentioned in the Minutes except statistically and occasionally when there was a complaint. The Chairman said at the Annual Meeting in 1859 that he believed that good feeding and good nursing were more conducive to getting patients out of hospital than anything else. Formerly there were many double beds. Now there was not one. But this meant less accommodation was available.

Up to now there has been no information about the number of nurses in the Hospital. In 1859 figures were published. There had been one nurse to twelve patients in 1834–35, one nurse to ten patients in 1844–45, and one to eight-and-a-half in 1858–59. This meant that there were about 15 nurses for 178 beds in 1834–35, 19 nurses for 191 beds in 1844–45 and 33 nurses for 277 beds in 1858–59. In 1968 there were 530 nurses for 516 available beds. There are so many more nursing activities these days, including theatres, casualty and out-patients, compared to a hundred years ago, but so far as ward work is concerned there are now 279 nurses for 516 beds. The salaries varied from £1 10s. to £6 5s. a quarter. Miss Owtram received 70 guineas per annum. There was one male nurse. The wards were apt to be unhealthy. Surgical wounds poured pus. Linseeed poultices were much in vogue; £200 a year was spent on this alone. The amount reached £308 in 1858 and the Board called for economy. The minutes have an interesting sidelight on the matter:

> Martha Mowbray who has been occupied in this Hospital for nearly twenty years in some of its most disagreeable work, that of removing the poultices from the surgical patients, and being by age and some infirmity incapacitated for continuing the duty, it appears to this Board not undesirable to make her some small weekly allowance to save her from destitution, she having no friends to assist her and no resources whereon she could rely for subsistence. Resolved that the sum of half-a-crown a week be allowed to her until this order be rescinded.

There was a new rule for the Matron made in 1861:

> The Matron shall, subject to the direction and approval of the Resident Medical Officer hire and discharge all the female servants and house porters and in like manner direct the whole household economy including the kitchens, wash houses and laundries and especially attend to the cleaning of the whole hospital and shall see that all the departments are conducted with regularity and economy.

On February 22, 1864, a letter was read from the Manchester and Salford Sanitary Association, whose Chairman, Thomas Turner, was one of the hospital's most distinguished surgeons, suggesting the advantages of establishing in Manchester a training school and home for nurses where women should be trained for the following purposes: (1) To serve as nurses in hospitals and other public institutions in the neighbourhood; (2) To be hired as sick nurses in private families; (3) To act as district or parish nurses amongst the poor. Practical instruction should be given in the wards of a large hospital, in particular the Royal Infirmary. The wheels turned slowly and it was not until the following September that a number of gentlemen interested in the establishment of an institution for the training of nurses in Manchester met in the Hospital Board Room.

The Board was asked for its views on the subject.. The Medical Committee thought the plan 'too comprehensive to be undertaken by the Medical Officers of the Infirmary until a preliminary and more simple system had been put into operation and specially applied to nurses already doing duty in the hospital wards'.

As a beginning, application was made to the Devonshire House Institution in London for 'a trained nurse whose duties would consist of teaching the Infirmary nurses all those details which are at present considered necessary to constitute efficiency and who will dine with the nurses and others and generally superintend them'. The Lady Superintendent of the Institution in London agreed to send one of her most experienced sisters 'thoroughly qualified in training others' and 'carrying a degree of *kind* authority in her manner' which was a very necessary qualification. It was suggested that she should come for six months at a salary of one guinea a week. The Resident Medical Officer was sent to London to interview her. He reported that the Lady Superintendent could not nominate a Lady Nurse who would be equal to the task of organising the nursing staff, but he had seen a very desirable person who had received a thorough training. It was agreed that she should be secured subject or otherwise, as after events may indicate, to the appointment of a Lady Nurse who would be head of the entire staff. This meant that the office of Matron had to be abolished.

Part 11

The Sister Superintendents

6

Mrs. Alice Walton 1865-66
Miss G. Henna 1867-71
Miss E. Darby 1871-76
Miss A. Dannatt 1876-78

The 'desirable person', Mrs. Walton, arrived from London in February 1865 to reorganise the whole system of training. She was not for several months in complete charge, for Miss Owtram was still Matron. But on June 22 it was made clear there was no longer a Matron, her office being abolished in consequence of the establishment in the hospital of the system of employing trained nurses under the general supervision of the House Stewards. The Chairman, at the Annual Meeting, welcomed the change and believed it would be beneficial to the patients. The hiring of nurses as in the past did not result in the same kind of attention being given to the patients as was expected under the new system.

There had to be changes in the rules. The appointment and dismissal of the nurses now rested with the Resident Medical Officer, who was to draw up such regulations as he thought fit, provided they were approved by the Medical Board and House Stewards. The Sister Superintendent would have under the direction of the Resident Medical Officer the general control of the nurses and wards and be responsible to him for the proper observance of the regulations.

The new rules meant that the Sister Superintendent was no longer responsible for supervising the cleaning of the whole hospital but only those departments under her charge. She no longer had the general control of the day and night nurses, and no longer had the power of suspending them instantly for misconduct. Nor was she responsible for seeing the nurses attended Divine Service, either in the Chapel or elsewhere. She no longer had to visit each patient to see that he was being properly looked after and receiving the correct diet. She was not responsible for seeing that nurses, who could be spared, should assemble at 8 p.m. in the Servants' Hall for scripture reading. She no longer had the power to appoint and dismiss nurses.

On November 17, 1865, a letter was received from the Manchester Nurse Training Institution and signed by a prominent member of the Infirmary Board. It stated that 'five of the eight Nightingale probationers at present undergoing instruction in nursing at St. Thomas's Hospital, London, were expected to return to Manchester on January 1'.

They were placed at the disposal of the Infirmary authorities with the hope that one or two wards might be assigned to them where they could carry out the system of nursing in which they had undergone a course of training. It was also hoped that the Board would institute training facilities so that nurses could be sent to private families.

The Board replied that such training facilities already existed. 'There were now seven nurses in attendance in private families' and the reports on their conduct had been most satisfactory. 'With regard to the offer of the services of the five nurses, the Board presumes that the two who were sent from the Infirmary, on the understanding that they were to return, are included in that number. They could make arrangements for the reception of the other three on receiving a fortnight's notice that they would be willing to enter the service of the Infirmary on the same terms and under the same regulations as the present nursing staff.' The Nightingale School of Nursing had started at St. Thomas's Hospital in 1860.

March 5, 1866
Sarah Newell, head nurse in the men's surgical wards, being incapacitated by the state of her health from the further discharge of her duties, it was resolved that in consideration of her having satisfactorily served the hospital for upwards of thirty years as a nurse she should be awarded a pension of ten shillings a week.

November 5, 1866
The following testimonial was granted to Mrs. Walton:
This is to certify that Mrs. Walton since February 1865 has had charge of the nursing department of this hospital under the direction of the Resident Medical Officer and discharged the duties which devolved on her to the satisfaction of the Weekly Board.

Unfortunately the progress made does not seem to have been maintained for in 1868 the standard of nursing in the hospital came

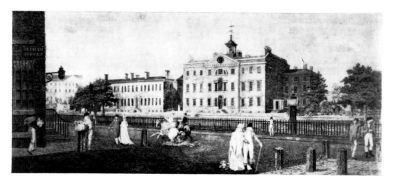

1 M.I. 1790

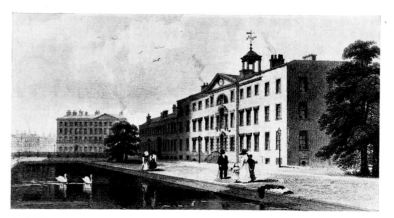

2 M.I. 1829

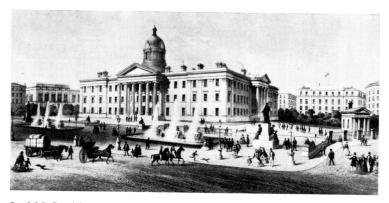

3 M.R.I. 1860

under review once again. With few exceptions the nine 'upper nurses' seemed to be efficient and trustworthy women. The 'under nurses', twenty-one in number, were on the whole not experienced enough for work in a large hospital, though many were skilled and intelligent. The eleven probationers were of little use in assisting the nurses or attending to the patients. They were only admitted for three months' training and this was nothing like sufficient. It was felt that the number of experienced nurses on the staff was not enough to justify the sending out of nurses to attend to patients in private families, and it was recommended 'that the whole supervision and control of the females throughout the establishment' be entrusted to a lady 'who could deal with all complaints and issue testimonials and certificates' and that the rules relating to the remuneration of the different orders of nurses be revised with the view of making the service more attractive and so retaining for a longer time women who prove themselves really efficient.

Miss G. Henna was appointed Sister Superintendent and arrived on April 29, 1867. She stayed until 1871 or thereabouts. Unfortunately the Wages Ledger is missing for this period and there was no mention of nursing in the Board minutes.

There were important happenings in the world of surgery. Joseph Lister had published the astonishing results of operating in an atmosphere of carbolic acid generated by a heated spray. This was the start of antiseptic surgery.

The first record of the use of Lister's methods in the Infirmary can be found in the operation register for January 28, 1870, when Mr. Lund removed a fatty tumour from a woman's back using 'Lister's carbolic plaster'. The next record of its use is in the following April for the excision of a knee joint. Both patients did well. The word antiseptic was first used in June 1871 when Mr. Lund and Mr. Dumville working together performed an amputation at the ankle: 'Wound treated antiseptically.' Thereafter the antiseptic method was freely used, but it was not until September 2, 1871, that an operation was performed in an atmosphere of carbolic acid generated by a spray. On that day Mr. Lund operated on an old fracture-dislocation of an elbow. 'Operation performed under carbolic acid spray. Wound dressed with carbolised muslin.' The wound healed in three weeks. In 1875 the Board approved of the suggestion that antiseptic dressings be provided for in-patients and out-patients. Lund, when he died, earned this benediction from the Board: 'He early recognised, practised and inculcated those antiseptic methods

D

inaugurated by Lord Lister, which have practically revolutionised surgical science to the lasting benefit of suffering humanity.'

There was a most regrettable occurrence about this time. Students were attending in increasing numbers and occasionally getting into trouble. In 1872 the Board was solemnly informed that one of them, Mr. Davies, had 'induced two nurses to go with him to a place of amusement.' The Board felt that it could not pass over such an occurrence as the students associating with the nurses either in or out of the Infirmary. It felt bound to inflict upon Mr. Davies as well as upon the nurses some deterrent sentence. Mr. Davies was pro-hibited from entering the Infirmary for three months and, in addi-tion, lost the session in which the offence was committed. It is not recorded what happened to the nurses, but at least it is clear that Mr. Davies believed in safety in numbers.

Miss E. Darby became Sister Superintendent when Miss Henna left, but there is no note of the date. Whole years go by without any mention of nurses or patients at the Weekly Board meetings other than statistical details of patients and occasional complaints about the way in which some patient has been treated or not treated. For these the Board always had a full answer after due enquiry and no interest was taken in the wards so long as they were formally reported as being healthy.

At the Annual Meeting in 1872 complaint was made that the appointment of Matron had been suspended for seven years without any notice to that effect having been given. This was 'very indecent on the part of the Board'. The Chairman explained that the Board experienced great difficulty in finding a matron suited to their requirements – one to whom they could give the control and autho-rity which the rules ordained. Mr. T. Ashton suggested that the present rules should be put in the fire and new ones drawn up.

We know from the Wage Books that there were sixty nurses in 1873 drawing between £7 10s. and £2 10s. a Quarter. The one man nurse was paid £3 11s. 6d.

At the 1874 Annual Meeting the Chairman reported that the income received from the services of private nurses (£1,416 3s.) was an important item. This was a matter to which the attention of the Board had been given for some time past. It had been found desirable to attend very closely to the training of nurses for their special duties and the greatest proof of the value of what had been done was the appreciation which these nurses had met with in private families. He considered this was a boon not only to the persons who employed them, but to the nurses themselves and to the Institution. It was well known that one of the great difficulties in former times was the finding of trustworthy and professional nurses. It was the duty of the Board to find proper apartments for the nurses as the Institution would probably become a great school for the training of nurses for the city.

Miss Darby left at the end of September 1876. She was succeeded by Miss A. Dannatt, who took over her duties on October 1.

At the start of 1877 some interesting statistics were published. Barnes Convalescent Hospital had started work in 1875. A Sister Superintendent was in charge, receiving a salary of £30, rising to £35, per annum. Monsall Fever Hospital belonged to the Infirmary. It had opened in 1871. The Matron's salary was £50, rising to £60, per annum.

The nursing establishment was as follows:

	1875	1877	
M.R.I.	70*	73*	(*plus one male nurse)
B.C.H.	7	6	
Monsall	11	12	

The Administrative Organisation at the Infirmary was overhauled and the Weekly Board became known as the Infirmary Committee. The Nurses and servants were asked in 1877 if they would accept money payment in lieu of beer. Eighteen of the 69 nurses agreed. Each was given an allowance of £2 per annum. All engagements in future would be made on the understanding that beer would not be supplied. So far there has been no mention of the accommodation occupied by the Nurses, but in 1878 this came under review:

The Nurses' dormitories on the first and second floors are placed in the most frequented corridors. No arrangements are made for comfort or convenience such as W.C.'s, lavatories, bathrooms or division into small dormitories. The head nurses' rooms are unsuitable both as regards position and plan, being awkwardly shaped and badly situated for supervision.

In 1878 the number of nurses had been reduced to 64, while the number of patients had increased to 271, and in November there is a note that a disciplinary case amongst the nurses had been referred to the Lady Superintendent of the Nurses. Miss Dannatt had been promoted.

It was in that same year that Nurse Ethel Manson[1] arrived at the hospital as a fee-paying probationer. The only record we have of her is the payment on January 30, 1879, of her fee of £6 10s. (Cash Book p. 407) (Figure 4.) She is the most distinguished nurse ever trained at the Infirmary. She was born in 1857 the younger daughter of a Morayshire farmer. At the age of 21 she entered the Children's Hospital, Nottingham, as a paying probationer. She continued her training with us during the years 1878–79, but we do not know how long she stayed. She left to become a Sister at the London Hospital. At the early age of 24 her recognised ability secured her the post of Matron and Superintendent of Nursing at St. Bartholomew's Hospital, London. She resigned in 1887 to marry Dr. Gordon Fenwick.

She was now able to use her remarkable intellect and ability to organise the nursing profession in the country. She founded in 1887 the British Nurses' Association, the first organisation of professional women to receive the Royal Charter (1893), the Matron's Council of Great Britain and the National Council of Nurses of Great Britain. She edited *The British Journal of Nursing* almost to her death at the age of 90.

But Mrs. Gordon Fenwick's most important work was her leadership of the movement for the State Registration of Nurses in spite of strong and active opposition from Florence Nightingale. She believed that Registration would largely abolish 'bad nurses'. Once giving evidence before a Parliamentary Select Committee[2] she told of a nurse who had trained at the London Hospital and went from there to Bart's, where she tried to poison a Sister with rat poison. She was quietly got rid of and next appeared on the staff of a nursing institute at Sheffield, where she was accused of poisoning a patient. She was tried at Leeds but escaped conviction through lack of evidence. She joined the nursing staff at the M.R.I. under an assumed name. While she was there three fires were started in the nurses' home and there were a large number of mysterious cases of poisoning among the patients. A detective was called in and eventually she was interviewed by a committee. She denied the incendiarism but admitted she was the nurse who had been tried at Leeds. She was dismissed but not prosecuted and the affair does not seem to appear

[1] *Dict. Nat. Biog.* 1941-50 p. 246

[2] 'Report from the Select Committee on Registration of Nurses, 1905,' May 11, 1904, p. 34.

in the hospital records. But as all names and dates were suppressed throughout, search has been hampered.

It took Mrs. Fenwick thirty-two years to succeed, for not until 1919 was the Nurses' Registration Act passed. She ranks very high in the hierarchy of political nurses. We are proud to have trained her. But all this lay in the future.

Part III

The Lady Superintendents of the Nurses

7

Miss A. Dannatt 1878-79
Miss K. Mackenzie 1879-80
Miss A. D. McKie 1881-86

Miss Dannatt was the first Lady Superintendent of the Nurses.

November 11, 1878
It was resolved that one ward could be set apart for four days at Christmas if it could be conveniently arranged for the purpose of private theatricals and that suitable suppers be provided afterwards. But no dancing was allowed.

In March 1879 the Secretary read correspondence from the Rev. G. S. Mitchell, a Catholic chaplain, who complained of the conduct of a Nurse who had desired him not to enter abruptly the female wards and had added that it was desirable that no male visitor should enter such wards without giving prior notice. The Committee ruled that the Nurse had acted correctly. This brought an offensive letter from the priest. The Committee stated that the tone of the letter precluded further correspondence but offered to meet him any Monday morning. He came and the matter was ironed out.

The question of the standard of nursing came up again in 1879. The present arrangements were unsatisfactory and needed a complete reorganisation. Nurses were frequently changed from ward to ward. There were too many partially instructed probationers compared to the number of properly qualified nurses. This was part of the trouble. But in addition there was want of sufficient direct supervision which the Head of the Nursing Staff ought to exercise over the details of nursing and the instruction of nurses. It was proposed to obtain the services of a lady thoroughly acquainted with practical duties of nursing and with the best methods of instructing nurses. The Lady Superintendent, Miss Dannatt, promptly resigned, giving three months' notice. Her resignation was accepted and the following advertisement was inserted in *The Times, The Lancet* and *The British Medical Journal:*

> Manchester Royal Infirmary. The post of Lady Superintendent of Nurses will shortly become vacant. The successful candidate must be thoroughly trained in all the duties of a practical nurse and familiar with the more modern systems of nursing organisation. Salary to commence at not less than one hundred guineas per annum with Board and Lodgings.

There were several applications and eventually it was decided to appoint Miss K. Mackenzie, then Lady Superintendent at the East London Hospital for Children. The Head Nurses, Agnes Naylor and Mrs. Mackin, were given a months' notice, the former being granted a pension of 10s. a week and the latter 10s. a week for three years. Both were allowed to stay on until the end of the year if they wished to do so. Head Nurse Rainforth acted as Superintendent for a month and was rewarded with a gratuity of three guineas.

The new Lady Superintendent at once asked that a Night Superintendent of Nurses be appointed at a salary of £35, and that the present practice of paying probationers their first remuneration after six months be abandoned. In future they should be paid quarterly. The Committee agreed at once to the first suggestion but deferred judgment on the second. It does not appear in the minutes again but must have been granted. Miss Mackenzie came forward with further suggestions in a letter dated November 22, 1879:

> This week I intend advertising in *The Lancet* the posts which will shortly be vacated through the departure of Mackin and Naylor. I should be very glad to know the Committee approves of my offering a little more salary with a view to commanding educated women to fill their places. I beg to submit the following rates at which the Sisters or Head Nurses are paid at some hospitals:
>
> | | |
> |---|---|
> | St. Thomas's | £35 |
> | London | £38 to £40 |
> | Guy's | £50 with nearly full board |
> | St. Bartholomew's | £60 partial board |
>
> I may mention that I consider £35 to £40 a fair salary.
>
> If it were the wish of the Board I should be glad to have their consent to introduce the name of 'Sisters' for the Heads of the Wards.
>
> Yours sincerely,
>
> K. Mackenzie,
> Lady Superintendent of Nurses.

The Committee agreed at once but there was a difficulty in obtaining Sisters from the Nightingale Home because beer was not allowed to nurses at the Infirmary and they required their travelling expenses. The Committee could not depart from the rule passed prohibiting the issue of beer to any nurse or servant, but they were willing to pay reasonable travelling expenses.

The staffing of the wards was next considered and it was agreed that there should be:

	Sisters	Staff Nurses
Men's Medical Wards	2	2
Women's Medical Wards	2	2
Men's Surgical Wards	3	3
Women's Surgical Wards	2	2
Total	9	9

The earliest register of nurses dates from Miss Mackenzie's arrival. It gives some interesting biographical details. The first entry and some other typical extracts are given below. It will be noted that a surprising number of nurses seem to have died at Monsall.

E. Brundrett. Engaged October 20, 1879. Would have made an excellent nurse. Her health failed after being here several months.

Annie Budrick. Engaged October 20, 1879. Has had women's surgical and male surgical as well as fever training. Towards the latter part of her stay here she has improved very much. Sent to Monsall. Dismissed for disobedience June 1881.

Ellen Hemming. Engaged November 1, 1879. Has been in male surgical and women's surgical, male medical and women's medical. Reports not so satisfactory as they ought to be. Sent to Monsall October 24. Dead.

M. Frost. Engaged November 13, 1879. Women's medical for over three months. Very moderate reports. Male surgical reports not very satisfactory. Male medical reports not so satisfactory as they ought to be. Night duty for several weeks in women's medical. She is conscientious and kind. Very slow. Sent to Monsall October 20, 1880. Male medical night duty March 3rd. Private staff April 1881. Makes an excellent private nurse. Has improved much in personal neatness. Is thoroughly conscientious and trustworthy. If not a brilliant nurse she is a *safe* one. Caught scarlet fever when in attendance on a private case and her health suffered so much that she was advised to take a situation abroad for a year. The Lady Superintendent obtained an appointment at San Remo for her and she left in October 1882. Re-engaged June 1883. Left to take private situation June 1884.

Alice Roberts. Engaged December 18, 1879. Three months male medical and well reported on. Three months in women's surgical (W.S.2) excellently reported on. Very obliging, interested in her work and keeps her patients very clean. Her marks for activity, method, thoroughness and ward management have been *very good*. Three months in male surgical – excellent reports. About two months on night duty in women's medical and did *very well*. December 10 sent to a private case. M.S.2. Staff Nurse March 1880. Did not succeed as a staff nurse. Was deficient in management and was not straightforward. Superseded September 1881. Private staff September 1881. Transferred herself to the service of her patient July 25, 1886 and therefore can never be re-engaged here and can have no reference. She knows this.

L. Newman. Engaged December 18, 1879. Male medical nearly three months. Very good reports. Male surgical over four months. *Very* satisfactory. A good nurse and always well reported on by her private patients. Inclined to be flighty in manner. Improved very much in 1882. Left for promotion as Head Nurse at Swansea June 12, 1882.

E. Tucker. Engaged January 1, 1880. A very fair private nurse, fond of her work and sparing no trouble over it. Has become capital nurse for smallpox and is much liked by Mr. Lund as a *very* good surgical nurse. Left to 'better herself' June 29, 1882.

Ellen White. Engaged February 14, 1880. Makes steady progress, excellent reports, kind and attentive to her patients and fond of her work. Sent to Monsall. Dead.

Francis Crowther. Engaged February 23, 1880. A quick, bright girl and a very fair nurse. Inclined to be flighty but improving. Dismissed for using bad language and striking a fellow nurse August 27, 1881.

Annie White. Engaged March 1, 1880. Dismissed as an utter failure as a nurse.

E. Lawton. Engaged March 25, 1880. Gets on well, cheerful, willing, very clean and tidy in her person and in all she does. An excellent nurse, general behaviour and conduct *very* good, a most upright and trustworthy woman. Left to 'better herself' July 3, 1883. Returned February 6, 1884. Made Sister of M.M.I. July 1884. Entirely satisfactory to staff and superintendent. July 1886.

M. Allen. Engaged April 15, 1880. Excellent reports, trustworthy and thoroughly reliable. Does exceedingly well. Left to 'better herself' May 1882. Re-engaged November 1882. Appointed Theatre Nurse January 1883. *Most* satisfactory July 1883. Left to be married Christmas 1884.

M. Beckett. Engaged May 3, 1880 – steady and trustworthy. A very fair nurse and daily improving. Always took tonsillitis when on ward duty so had to do private duty. Thoroughly satisfactory in every way. A most admirable private nurse. Has this nurse left?

A. McKean. Engaged May 15, 1880. Dismissed July 1881. A very indifferent nurse, stupid, dirty, untidy and conceited.

S. Whitelegge. Engaged July 7, 1880. Very good reports. Bright, active, intelligent and thorough. A very quick girl, clever, a good nurse, most willing and obliging. Contracted typhoid and died June 29, 1885.

L. Jefferson. Engaged July 28, 1880. Not very satisfactory. Neither kind nor trustworthy. Discharged July 1882.

E. Ball. Engaged August 4, 1880. Fairly satisfactory. Attentive to and interested in her work, manner often a little rough. Dismissed for going out without leave.

Emma Roberts. Engaged August 1880. Got on very well, very kind to the patients and obedient to the head of the ward. December 10 sent to Monsall. Dead.

S. Rossington. Engaged August 23, 1880. Interested in and attentive to her work, active, bright, attentive, obedient and generally good. Has excellent reports, orderly, very kind to her patients and generally promises to make a good nurse, a steady, modest girl. Left, giving notice on account of being married October 1884. This was not true. Should never be re-engaged.

Isabella Hinch. Engaged September 30, 1880. A sensible, trustworthy woman and a very good nurse. Promoted to Staff Nurse September 15, 1881 (within a year). An excellent nurse. Now a very good influence on her ward and is most loyal to the Sister. Appointed Sister on probabtion September 1883 (within 3 years of her induction). Surgeons and Lady Superintendent alike satisfied. An admirable Sister 1886. Gives complete satisfaction to the staff and manages her lobby remarkably well.

Marian Greatorex. Engaged October 1880, indifferent in every way. Left December 1881. Advised to give up hospital nursing.

Lizzie Young. Engaged October 12. Quite unsuitable for a nurse being stupid, self-satisfied and clumsy. Dismissed July 1881.

Mary Ann Williams. Engaged November 20, 1880. Refused to go to Monsall. Dismissed July 1881. Would have made a good nurse.

Elizabeth Jones. Engaged November 24 1880. Too young and giddy but a good willing worker. Dismissed.

Of the 50 nurses engaged in 1880, 15 made good, 20 were dismissed, 6 died, 2 failed in health, 1 left to be married, 3 left to better themselves and 3 resigned. Here are some reasons for dismissal: 'health failed' (there are a lot of similar notes). 'Left as she was not allowed to take a fortnight's holiday as she desired – never to be re-engaged having been very troublesome of late – hysterical,' 'dismissed for theft,' 'broke her engagement in an unfair way and left,' 'temper again troublesome – served here under a false name,' 'not strong enough,' 'by no means satisfactory – dismissed – serious rumours against her moral character have since been heard,' 'ran away' (she wasn't the only one to do so), 'dismissed for over familiarity with the male patients,' 'dismissed for neglect of a patient,' and 'dismissed for flighty conduct.'

In 1878 it was regarded as essential that a Nurses' Home should be built. This would enable the Board not only to provide sufficient healthy and detached sleeping accommodation for the nursing staff, but would render the retention of wooden sheds unnecessary. Unfortunately there was no money available for building and the nurses had to sleep in the huts. There was no room for them in the main building. There were at that time 91 nurses at the Infirmary. Five were paid £30 a year, one £26, three £22, twenty £20, fourteen £18, nineteen £15, twenty-nine £12, one £100 (presumably the Lady Superintendent), and nine scrubbers one shilling a day. It was said that nurses had to get up at 6 o'clock in the morning and spend two hours doing housemaids' work scrubbing the floors of their wards before beginning the work of day nurses, and it was asked whether it was right to put refined ladies to such hard and menial work.

Miss Mackenzie seems to have resigned in the Autumn of 1880. There is a minute dated October 18 dealing with the interviewing of candidates for the vacancy. On November 16 it was decided to appoint Miss Agnes Dunlop McKie as from January 1, 1881. The Board expressed their gratitude by resolving that on the retirement of Miss Mackenzie (now Mrs. Hayward), the Lady Superintendent of Nurses, after faithful and satisfactory services, the thanks of the Committee are hereby tendered to her with best wishes for her future happiness.

On the same day plans for the building of a Nurses' Home were considered. It was to accommodate 72 nurses. There seems to be a discrepancy here in view of the number of nurses just recorded. Two members of the Board were appointed to inspect their sleeping accommodation with power to subdivide the rooms as they might consider necessary in order to secure more privacy.

The charges for private nurses were increased to 31s. 6d. a week and to two guineas a week for infectious patients. Payment one week in advance was required. Six hundred and twenty-five twill sheets were bought at 1s. 2d. a yard.

Plans for the Nurses' Home were submitted to the Medical Board. It was agreed that the night nurses should be provided with separate bedrooms. Building began in 1882.

Miss McKie was soon making improvements. A Home Sister was appointed at a salary of £40 per annum. Her own salary was increased to £150 from September 29 in view of the increased duties and responsibilities which would devolve on her upon the opening of the Nurses' Home.

The new Nurses' Home was brought into use in December 1882, being occupied by its full complement of nurses. No plans were made for an increase of staff. The 77 nurses each had a separate bedroom. There were apartments for the Lady Superintendent, the Home Sister (who had charge of the building), 8 head nurses or sisters, 12 staff nurses, 27 probationers, 17 night nurses, 8 private nurses who were willing to receive engagements in private families, and three nurses who might have 'the misfortune to be disabled through sickness from performing their duties'. The cost of building, furniture and fittings was £5,780. It consisted of three floors and was connected to the hospital by a covered way communicating with the first floor. Each bedroom contained about a thousand cubic feet of space and was furnished with a bed, a lavatory basin, a fixed mirror, a falldown writing table and a good-sized wardrobe. The floors were stained and varnished and the furniture and fittings were of pitch pine. Each floor was provided with a good-sized general room for the use of the nurses. That on the top floor was intended for a recreation and reading room. Through the kindness of some ladies it was furnished with a piano. The general room on the second floor was a library and reading room and that on the ground floor a workroom for sewing. Each floor contained two bathrooms with hot and cold water and the building was heated by steam coils.

The new Nurses' Home seems to have put a strain on the Lady Superintendent for in 1883 she was given two months' leave of absence to recover her health. Shortly after it was decided to give the nurses a trip to the country, the details being left to the General Superintendent and Miss McKie.

In 1883 it was reported that Sister Harbord had wilfully disobeyed an order from the General Superintendent, sent by telegram, to return to the Infirmary on the 9th instant, which she admitted she had received. She had been given leave of absence to the 8th, but did not return until the 11th. Her explanation was most unsatisfactory. She refused to remain under suspension but preferred to leave the Infirmary without delay. The Committee thought that this was most desirable under all the circumstances.

There were complaints about the frequency with which the Nurses were employed in attendance on various members of the Medical Staff at operations and in the wards during the dinner-time from 12-30 to 1 p.m. The importance of the due attention to the distribution of dinner to the patients promptly and efficiently was dwelt upon. The Infirmary Committee asked the Medical Board to give this question their consideration. The Medical Board recognised the expediency of carrying the suggestion into effect as far as possible.

There was trouble too because a nurse named E. Hall, whom Miss McKie had dismissed some months ago, had been engaged at Monsall Fever Hospital, which was still part of the Infirmary, without any reference to her. The Committee referred the matter to the Monsall Committee saying that if the facts were correct she should be dismissed.

In 1882 Miss McKie was granted one month's leave of absence. In the same year Certificates of Efficiency were granted to Sisters Eleanor Farnworth, Sarah Burkhill, Eliza Davies, Isabella French, and Nurses Sarah Edwards, Louisa Plunket, Elizabeth Nelson and Robina Ferguson. The Chairman of the Medical Board was asked to sign them on behalf of the examiners. This was a new venture.

A new problem arose in 1885. The Medical Officer of Health attended a meeting of the Infirmary with respect to the conveyance of Infirmary Nurses in cabs from private cases of an infectious nature. It was decided that in future a rule should be printed on the form used when sending a nurse out to a private case to the effect that in cases of infectious disease it was incumbent upon an employer to cause the nurse to be disinfected before leaving his house, and also that a printed slip be sent with each nurse going to an infectious case to be handed by her to the medical attendant requesting him to kindly ascertain that the foregoing precaution has been carried out. This was later amended. The nurse on leaving the case must take a bath and put on clean clothes. The infected clothes should be put in a closed box to be carried on top of the conveyance containing the nurse and sent to be disinfected.

A form of certificate of proficiency granted to nurses after examination was approved. These were to be signed by the Lady Superintendent and the Chairman of the Medical Board. The examination of nurses now became a regular procedure twice a year.

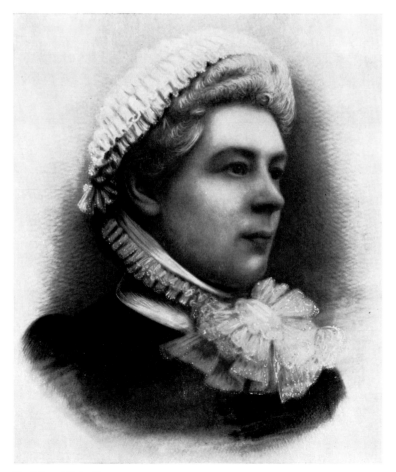

4 Nurse Manson's fee

5 Miss Alicia Browne

Miss McKie was given leave of absence in consequence of ill-health in January 1886. On May 3 she resigned her appointment and requested to be relieved of her duties on August 5. An advertisement was immediately issued, salary £100 per annum with board and lodging. It was a sad loss for she got on well with both lay and medical boards and was well liked by her nurses and the patients. She married an Edinburgh doctor, Graham Steell, who eight years earlier had joined the Infirmary staff as Resident Medical Officer and became one of its most distinguished physicians. She made him a good wife. Some of her nurses visited her annually and several became well known Sisters, among them Sister Stephens, the legendary Sister Reid (her husband's ward sister), Sister Slinger and Sister Arthur. Miss McKie died in 1910. We were then told she had come to Manchester from Glasgow Royal Infirmary and had worked persistently to raise the standard and tone of nursing.

E

8

Miss Alicia Browne 1886-91

Miss Browne was elected Lady Superintendent on June 11, 1886, and presumably took over her duties the following August. Within a year she almost lost the services of her Home Sister, Miss Stone, who asked the Committee for a testimonial as she was applying for another post, and was given one expressive of their approval of the way she had performed her duties during the past four years. In July the nurses were given a one-day trip into the country or to the seaside at the expense of the Institution. Later in the year they were each given a cape made of baize or other warm material as an addition to their uniform.

Miss Browne's salary was increased from £100 to £150 per annum in December 1887, and about the same time she did really lose the services of Miss Stone on the grounds of ill-health. She was granted a gratuity of six months' salary (£20).

Early in 1888 the Medical Superintendent of Guy's Hospital asked if the Committee would be prepared to co-operate in the adoption of a scheme for the registration of qualified nurses. The Committee declined, but did not give any reason for refusal. This must have been the British Nurses' Association founded by our own Mrs. Gordon Fenwick, an organisation that tried hard to improve the standard of nursing but never got the support it deserved, although it won the Royal accolade. More will be heard about it in Chapter 10.

The comfort of the patients was improved in 1888 by the withdrawal of straw mattresses from the wards. They were replaced by woven wire mattresses and silent castors were fixed to all beds. The question of employing ladies as nurses was discussed at a meeting of the Board of Governors in 1889.

Mr. A. Simpson moved in accordance with notice – 'That the instructions given to the Lady Superintendent of Nurses to decline all applications as nurses from those who ought to be described as ladies, be withdrawn.'

Mr. W. J. Crossley seconded the motion and after much discussion the question was adjourned for a week. At the next meeting the discussion was resumed. – Mr. A. Neild moved an amendment. 'That the Chairman, Secretary, and Lady Superintendent be requested to report to the committee whether there is in force any rule, expressed or implied, which fetters the discretion of the Lady Superintendent in engaging women of superior education as nurses.' The amendment and motion were lost.

Mr. Simpson, referring to these minutes, said that in addition to the regulations under which the Lady Superintendent at present admitted nurses he understood that there had been an instruction given which was not written, by which the Lady Superintendent had no option but to refuse the application for admission as a nurse from a person who would be described as a lady. He thought there should have been no alteration whatever. He was conscious that in excluding those to whom he had referred they were depriving their patients of the services of a body of women specially qualified and whose services would be specially acceptable to their patients. He believed the main, if not the sole, objection of the committee to the adoption of his resolution was with regard to the Matron's discipline in the hospital, and that some difficulty might arise in sending out nurses in private families. If other hospitals larger than theirs circumstanced precisely the same as regards their patients and their private nurses, found by practice that ladies when admitted were amenable to discipline as nurses and performed their work as other nurses did and those hospitals benefited thereby, he asked why they should deprive their patients of similar advantages merely on the ground of anticipating difficulties in the maintenance of discipline and the sending out of private nurses.

Mr. Alfred Neild said he thought that to throw any obstruction in the way of lady nurses was a very grave matter, and he was sorry that the resolution of the committee had tended to do that. He could not believe that what was done in other hospitals was impossible in the Manchester Infirmary. There was no doubt that women came as ladies who were utterly unsuitable, but such failures were not general. There was, however, much ambiguity about the term 'ladies'. If it meant simply ladies of good family who wished to go to the Infirmary to amuse themselves he objected to lady nurses, but if by ladies they meant women of good education and gentle bringing up, but who had to earn their bread, he thought anything which tended to shut them out when they were willing to conform to the rules was a most disastrous thing in the interests of the patients.

Alderman King said he thought it was rather to be regretted that the decision of the House Committee which had been arrived at after great care and consideration should be again discussed. An obvious duty rested upon the committee, and it was difficult for the members always to give public expression to their reasons for a special course of action. The committee had acted with a desire for the best interests of the institution. Many ladies, no doubt, would be useful as nurses, but nothing could be better than the present system of nursing at the Infirmary, about which universal satisfaction was expressed. They were doing well now, and there was no need for further change.

Mr. Neild said the Board had at least the right to discuss the work of committee.

The chairman said the committee felt that to make a needless change in arrangements which were giving very great satisfaction would be an unwise step, and that if the proposed change were made they would run the risk of encountering difficulties from which they are now happily entirely free. The presence of ladies on the private nursing staff, which was now bringing in to them splendid reports, and on which in the ordinary course of duty they would have to serve, would be a most serious difficulty, as there were ladies who did not like to be attached to this service, and in some families their presence would be a source of serious embarrassment.

The minutes referred to were passed without further comment.

There were two deaths among the nursing staff. The night superintendent and sister, Eleanor Farnworth, contracted diphtheria from a patient. She had been a nurse and a sister for nine years and 'had given very faithful service.' Miss Agnes Naylor, late Head Nurse until 1880, died in 1889. She had been receiving a pension of ten shillings a week. Pensions for Nurses came under review in 1891. Any nurse who could produce evidence of having attained the age of 50 years and who had been not less than 25 years in continuous service to the hospital and who should be, in the opinion of the Board of Management, unfit for further work and of satisfactory character would receive a pension of £25 per annum, payable quarterly. If any nurse of not less than 10 years' service should, from no fault of her own, break down in health to such an extent as to render her unfit for further work, the Board, on being furnished with satisfactory medical evidence, might award her such pension, gratuity or allowance (temporary or otherwise) as they thought proper. The Board reserved the right to discontinue any such pension or allowance if they considered it desirable from any cause. A pension would be liable to forfeiture in case of misconduct or any other cause which in the opinion of the Board might render a pensioner no longer a fit object to enjoy such pension.

On July 6, 1891, Miss Browne resigned as from September 25, 1891. The Committee accepted it 'with great regret' and an advertisement was issued – salary £100 per annum with board and lodging.

Up to now every member of the nursing staff has been faceless and there has been no mention of character. In fact, the minutes of Lay and Medical Boards run on for years without any reference to them. There might have been no nurses in the hospital. But there is a portrait in colour of Miss Browne (Figure 5). It shows a good-looking, placid, blue-eyed, grey-haired woman in a black blouse with a very frilly white cap and what almost looks like a ruff round her neck tied with a large frilly bow. On the back are some biographical details. 'Born in 1851, she entered Barts when she was 30, became a sister there in 1881. Five years later she came to Manchester. She left the Infirmary to join the All Saints Sisterhood, and later became Matron of New Somerset Hospital, Capetown, which they staffed. She died on June 28, 1934.' Her retirement paved the way for one of the best Matrons the Infirmary ever had.

9

Miss Florence M. Calvert 1891-1907

The appointing committee met on August 4, 1891, and appointed Miss Florence Calvert Lady Superintendent. She was well known to them for she was Matron at the Monsall Fever Hospital.

Soon after the appointment Sister Catherine Gaynor applied for a pension on completion of 25 years' service, and being over 50 years of age and unfit to work she was granted a pension of £25 per annum.

Miss Calvert began very wisely by looking into the training arrangements of her nurses. She asked for a new skeleton for their instruction, and then through the Infirmary Committee the Medical Board were requested to nominate annually two of their number to deliver a course of lectures to Nurses on medical and surgical nursing, and for this instruction an honorarium of one guinea a lecture was suggested. The Medical Board was also requested to prepare a syllabus of such lectures. Dr. Wilkinson and Mr. Thorburn were nominated as lecturers. Satisfactory attendance at the lectures was compulsory.

Certificates of efficiency were regularly being presented to nurses who had passed an examination. But now prizes of the value of two and one guinea were awarded to Nurses Bullough and Brenner. Clearly there was a good pass standard required, for three nurses failed to satisfy the examiners and were referred to further examination at the end of six months.

There was correspondence in *The Courier* in 1893 concerning nurses' grievances. Although the criticisms were denied, as will be seen, by two members of the nursing staff, it seems likely that there must have been some truth in the complaints. The following letter was signed 'A Sympathiser with Nurses."

There is one institution of which Mancunians are proud but I feel assured that if the public were aware of the cruel manner – for the treatment amounts to cruelty – in which nurses at the Manchester Royal Infirmary are treated they would insist upon a complete alteration of the system, not only on behalf of the nurses, but for the sake of the patients who are under their care. To enter into details would take up too much of your space, but I will touch upon some of the points that appear most prominently to need reform. That the probationers or day nurses should not be required to scour the floors of the wards, the cupboards, and other menial work of that kind which they at present have to do instead of attending to the patients, and that they should receive some practical instruction in matters relating to their profession, instead of being left to pick up such knowledge as they can promiscuously. That more time should be allowed in which the nurses can give the patients their dinner. A nurse may have 18 patients to attend to, their dinners are ready about half an hour before the dinner hour of the nurses, and the nurse has to bring into the ward each patient's dinner. She may have two, three, or four patients whom she has to feed, and she must have all their dinners finished and be herself down in the nurses' dining hall at the prescribed hour. If she fail she will be reprimanded and reported: consequently she is compelled to make the patients take their food as quickly as they can swallow it. This cannot be good for the patients. The food provided for the nurses should be properly cooked, and decently served. At present the idea seems to be that anything in the way of cooking is good enough for the nurses, and the tea and coffee are made almost nauseous, not from the fault of the quality of either, but by the manner in which they are prepared. The pity is that there is nobody to take any interest in the comfort of the nurses, and any complaint made would receive no attention, but would probably cause a prejudice against the person complaining. The day nurses come on duty in the wards at 7 a.m., and for the first two hours are working at top pressure in scouring and cleaning the wards. They go to dinner at one o'clock, and are supposed to go out for exercise for two hours in the afternoon, either from two till four or from four till six. They have tea and come on duty till nine o'clock, when they go to supper, and after supper they have to attend service in the chapel. All the time they are on duty they are not allowed to sit down or rest in any way, so that by the time they go off duty (after 9 p.m.) it may be imagined they are tired out; but tired or not, whether their feet and limbs ache through long hours of standing, they must attend chapel and sing hymns. Picture the mockery of it; keeping people without any practical rest the whole day, and then require them to take part in religious exercises, when, as is frequently the case, they are suffering actual pain from sheer fatigue. Would any medical man allow any person he cared for to be on their feet for so many hours daily as are the probationers at the Manchester Royal Infirmary? In the factories, where the work is much lighter and is not attended with the responsibilities that are inseparable from nursing the sick, the law forbids the employment of women for more than a certain number of hours – even though they may actually desire to continue working. Surely some steps ought to be taken – (a) to shorten the hours of duty; (b) to provide for proper instruction, at all events, for newcomers, and (c) for the proper cooking and serving of the meals. I have said nothing of the night nurses, but as I have trespassed so far I will conclude with the hope that these lines may induce some persons who have the power to use their influence in the direction stated above.

'Paris' replied as follows:

Having trained at the Manchester Royal Infirmary, I cannot express the indignation I felt on reading the 'Sympathiser with Nurses' ' letter on the treatment of nurses at that institution. Having only left it a few months, I cannot think things have so changed as to necessitate the nurses scouring the ward floors, which are all polished. If a nurse cannot clean out a small cupboard and help to keep the ward in order without putting it in the papers, she is not fit for a nurse. All nurses know there is a certain amount of hard work to do the first year, and it must be gone through, or how can we expect to be able to train nurses ourselves if we are not thoroughly acquainted with all the minor details of ward work? Provided a nurse has 18 patients' dinners to see after, they are all put on a tray by the sister; nurse has only to give them round the ward, and as a rule the staff nurse feeds the helpless patients, they certainly are not left to the tender mercy of young probationers. I can also say nurses are not allowed to pick up what little knowledge they can themselves; but are thoroughly and practically trained in all branches of nursing. As regards the time on duty, it is no longer than in any other large hospital, and the time off much better, considering they have a day every month. Surely any nurse cannot grumble at giving 15 minutes to prayers. It may be a mockery to some, but I hope not to all. As for the nurses' comforts, what more can they want than a good home, a kind matron and home sister to look after them? And these they have. Perhaps it would be as well if the 'Sympathiser' would take his own and nurses' friends to some of the factories he thinks so superior to the Manchester Royal Infirmary, and not give an opinion on matters they evidently know little or nothing about. As a Manchester nurse, I am sorry to think there are some who have so little respect for themselves or confidence in their superior officers as to have to carry their grievances to the papers. That I thought was a privilege reserved for London nurses only.

There was also a reply from 'A Probationer':

I write on behalf of a number of my sister nurses who have just finished our first year of probationer's duty. During that time we have always found our superiors in office most ready to train us, sympathise with us and help us in any possible way. I take it your correspondent defines the word 'train' as a systematic drumming of the theoretical part of nursing but any sensible person will agree that 'training' in the sense which nurses require it embraces habits of order, cleanliness, gentleness and quietness, without these the theoretical training would be worth nothing and no true woman would object to scouring provided it is for the good of the patients. No work of whatever kind and no woman possessed of any refinement of feeling would deem it degrading.

Finken versus the Manchester Royal Infirmary

In 1893 Miss Finken – a discharged nurse – entered an action in the Queen's Bench division of the High Court of Justice against the Institution. She was given an opportunity of attending the Board of Management on November 1, 1893, to explain the circumstances under which she returned from Lymm on November 25, 1892. But the case went on.

The action took place at the Assizes before Mr. Justice Day on November 10, 1893. The evidence was as follows: Nurse Finken had been sent with another nurse to deal with an outbreak of small-pox at Lymm. The other nurse took ill and Nurse Finken had to work day and night in very unhygienic and distressing conditions. Miss Calvert asked that the sick nurse should be sent back to the Infirmary as soon as she was fit to travel. Nurse Finken, who by now was far from well, returned at the same time. Both were sent to Monsall Fever Hospital, where Nurse Finken was found to have a temperature of 103.8. No diagnosis was made, but she recovered and was sent home for some sick leave. On her return she was asked why she had left the small-pox patient's house, and on replying that she felt ill, she was told that she had no right to leave her patients and because she had done so she was 'a disgrace to the hospital' and must take a month's notice to leave. Nurse Finken reminded Miss Calvert that she had given satisfaction to the hospital and that in private cases her reports had been uniformly complimentary. She asked leave to sit her examination. Miss Calvert refused her this privilege and would not allow her to appeal to the Board of Management.

The Judge expressed an opinion to the effect that the regulations signed on engagement by the Plaintiff entitled her at the expiration of three years of admittedly satisfactory service as a Nurse to present herself for examination by a Committee of the Medical Board, and if she satisfied the examiners to receive a certificate of efficiency.

The Counsel for the Infirmary (Mr. Gully, Q.C., M.P.) consented to the issue of a mandamus with costs. The Medical Board were requested to arrange for the examination of Miss L. A. Finken for her nursing certificate early in January 1894. She was duly examined and with two other nurses awarded her certificate.

New Regulations for the Engagement and Training of Nurses

Miss Calvert for some time had discussed with the Board the regulations she desired for the engagement and training of nurses. These 'New Regulations for the Engagement and Training of Nurses' were approved by the Board of Management on February 26, 1894, and duly printed.

1. Women, who must be unmarried, or widows, are received for training in the Manchester Royal Infirmary, between the ages of 25 and 35. They must be well educated; and they will be required to produce satisfactory references as to character, and a medical certificate of good health. Personal application must be made to the Lady Superintendent of Nurses at the Hospital, between 10 and 12 a.m.

2. After a month's trial (for which period they do not receive wages or uniform), and on being approved, they will be expected to remain in the service of the Infirmary for three years. They will be subject to dismissal, however, at any time, in case of misconduct, or if they should be considered inefficient, or are inattentive to their duties. After the completion of the period of probation, which may, at the discretion of the Lady Superintendent of Nurses, extend over two years, they will be employed in the Infirmary, on the Private Nursing Staff (either in private families or in other Hospitals), or at the Convalescent Hospital, Cheadle, as the Lady Superintendent may direct.

3. Probationers will act as Assistant Nurses in the Wards of the Hospital. They will be instructed in their duties by the 'Sisters' (Head Nurses), who will report every month to the Lady Superintendent as to the manner in which they perform their various duties.

4. They will also receive Theoretical Instruction from Members of the Honorary Staff of the Hospital, who deliver courses of Lectures to the Nurses on Medical and Surgical Nursing during each year.

5. Nurses, after the completion of three years' continuous service, and who are recommended by the Lady Superintendent of Nurses as having passed satisfactorily through the prescribed course of training and instruction, will be examined in the months of January or July by a Committee of the Medical Board, if then in the employment of the Infirmary, and, if reported qualified, will be given Certificates of efficiency and good conduct as Trained Nurses.

6. The following is the scale of payment, with board, laundry, and medical attendance, which will be given to Nurses if engaged at the expiration of their month's trial: 1st year, £10; 2nd year, £15; 3rd year, £18; 4th year, £20. After which the increase will be £1 annually up to a maximum of £25. *Certificated* Trained Nurses, while employed on the Private Nursing Staff, will receive in addition to the above scale of wages, the sum of £5 per annum. Nurses on the Private Nursing Staff also receive one-half of the extra charge of 10s. 6d. per week made for each infectious or massage case nursed by them.

7. Uniform dress – consisting of 3 print dresses, 8 aprons, and 3 caps – is given to each Probationer at the expiration of her month's trial, and is renewed yearly. In the event of a Nurse or Probationer leaving the Infirmary, from any cause, before the expiration of 12 months from date of last issue of her Uniform its estimated value will be deducted from her wages. The Nurses are expected to wear their Uniform on all occasions when they are on duty. They must provide their own outdoor dress, which should be plain and neat.

8. Nurses must give one calendar month's notice before leaving the service of the Hospital, and will receive the same from the Lady Superintendent; but, in case of misconduct, neglect of duty, or wilful disobedience, they will be liable to instant dismissal.

9. Nurses will be allowed sixteen days' leave of absence every year. They will also be give a day's holiday every month, provided the Lady Superintendent can arrange for this without inconvenience to the work of the Hospital. Nurses must not be absent themselves from the Hospital, nor from duty, without the permission of the Lady Superintendent.

10. The Nurses are under the authority of the Lady Superintendent, who is responsible for the observance of these regulations.

11. The Senior Nurses may, if eligible, be promoted to the higher rank of 'Sister' (Head Nurse), to whom special rates of payment and a distinctive Uniform are given.

12. Nurses of long and faithful service will be entitled to pensions.

N.B.—The expression 'Nurses', shall also include 'Head Nurses' and 'Probationers'.

The applicant had to agree to enter the service of the Manchester Royal Infirmary subject to the above Regulations, and to conform to the By-laws of the Institution in force from time to time. The pension regulations for Nurses remained as detailed in 1891.

In 1894 the General Superintendent submitted a return of the routine work on the wards between 5 a.m. and 10 p.m. He was instructed to send a copy to the Medical Board.

5 *a.m. to* 9 *a.m.* wash patients, make beds, clean and polish grates and floors, dust wards and tidy generally.

8 *a.m.* patients' breakfasts.

9 *a.m. to* 1-30 *p.m.* various ward rounds, massage, dressings, operations, etc.

12 *to* 1 *p.m.* dinner.

1 *to* 2 *p.m.* patients get up, beds made, wards tidied.

2 *to* 4-30 *p.m.* wards cleaned. Visiting day Thursday, 2–4 p.m.

4-30 *to* 5 *p.m.* tea.

5 *p.m. to* 8 *p.m.* wash patients, make beds, sweep and dust wards.

7-30 *p.m.* supper.

8 *p.m.* lights lowered.

9 *p.m. to* 10 *p.m.* Residents go round.

In 1894 Miss Calvert's salary was raised to £125 per annum. Next year a request was read from the Nursing Association, Derby, for the Board to accept Probationers who had had a year's training at Crumpsall Workhouse Infirmary and give them one year's training at the Manchester Royal Infirmary. The Committee were unable to comply, but they did agree to the suggestion made by the Medical Board that another Sister should be appointed to the Medical Wards when there was money available.

The question of moving the hospital to its present site came up for discussion in 1896 and plans were drawn up. The Medical Board were critical of several items, including (1) No Nurses' home was provided except the problematical one in 'three houses to be purchased in Nelson Street', (2) A Sister or Head Nurse had charge of 60 beds which was about twice the number she could efficiently manage.

The annual picnic for nurses was discontinued. Instead of this an extra day was added to their annual holiday.

The second Sister to be employed in the female medical wards was finally agreed upon and provision made for a sitting and bed-room combined by taking from the end of Queen Ward a similar space to that now occupied by the Ovarian Ward. It was also resolved that the suggestion of the Medical Board that accommodation for the private nurses be obtained outside the building was undesirable, and that unless a bedroom be provided as previously suggested they did not see their way to carry out the proposed addition to the nursing staff of the second Sister.

By 1898 Miss Calvert's salary had been increased from £125 to £150.

It is surprising to find in 1901 that the scheme of supplying citizens with private nurses had become less popular than it used to be. It was decided to draw up an advertisement setting forth the fact that there was a highly efficient staff of trained nurses at the Infirmary available at any time for the sick in private families at fixed rates of payment. The advertisement was placed twice weekly in the *Manchester Guardian* and on Saturdays in the *City News*.

It had been suggested that a masseur should be appointed and also a male nurse to look after uncontrollable cases. However, it was agreed to appoint a porter for the latter purpose and to accept the offer made by Mr. J. Allison of the Hydropathic establishment, Hyde Road, to supply when required a skilled masseur to massage cases at a charge of 1s. 6d. each a day up to four cases, and a shilling a day for any greater number for a period of three months.

The year 1902 brought a big change in the membership of the Committee. There had been an important meeting of subscribers to discuss the Committee's plan to rebuild and enlarge the Infirmary on its site in Piccadilly. This had been defeated and instead it had been decided to build a new hospital near the University. The Committee therefore resigned and a new one was elected. But at its last meeting the old committee passed resolutions of thanks to various members of the administrative staff, including this one:—

Of another prominent and valued officer, Miss F. M. Calvert, Lady Superintendent of Nurses, the committee wish to record their high estimate of long and useful service rendered to the Monsall Fever Hospital and latterly to the Royal Infirmary. Throughout the fourteen years during which Miss Calvert has held these appointments she has discharged the duties – often difficult and delicate, always important – to their entire satisfaction and this Committee welcomes the opportunity of offering their parting testimony to her remarkable capacity, amiability and unremitting devotion to the best interest of the Charity.

Miss Catherine Gaynor, a former Sister, died in 1903. She had been in receipt of an annual pension of £25 since October 1891. It is nice to know that the Board could increase the pension allowance in special circumstances. Nurse Gothard, who had only worked in the hospital for 18 years, was given a special pension of £20 a year in consequence of her serious ill-health, and Miss Arthur, the Home Sister, who had served for upwards of 30 years and was now bedfast, was granted £35 a year, an increase of £10.

In 1903 a Bill was brought to Parliament sponsored by the Royal British Nurses' Association advocating the Registration of Trained

Nurses. The Infirmary, with other hospitals, opposed it but no reason
was given for this decision.

The Medical Board in 1905 was of the opinion that the present
management of the operating theatres was a source of great danger.
The number of operations performed in a morning was very great and
the succession of cases had to be rapid. The requirements of modern
surgery called for most careful attention to detail on the part of all
concerned including sisters and nurses. Those who handled instruments should have no other duties of any kind. As things were the
theatre sister cleaned instruments, prepared douches and other im-
perfectly sterilised apparatus, handled patients' bed clothes and the
like and went from one theatre to the other attending to other minor
points. The confusion was very great, constituting a great source
of danger and much waste of time.

It was difficult to suggest a remedy which was practicable and
completely met the case, but an improvement would be effective if:
(1) Additional instruments (duplicates) were provided so that a
second series could be prepared efficiently without delay. (2) An
additional nurse was provided for each of the two theatres. (3) The
nurse assisting with the instruments should never have any duties
which rendered her hands septic. (4) These nurses should have con-
tinuity of service. The surgical staff did not consider that the nurses
as a whole were reliable in aseptic surgery, but feared that under
existing conditions of confusion it would not be possible to insist
upon the strict attention to detail that was essential. After some
discussion the Committee agreed to provide accommodation for the
two extra nurses.

New 'Regulations for the Engagement and Training of Nurses' were
drawn up and approved by the Board of Management on January 29,
1906, and show many changes from those of 1894.

1. There are two classes of Nurses :—
(a) Those undergoing training of less than three years' service and
uncertificated, and
(b) Those who are of more than three years' service and certificated.

2. *Regulations affecting Uncertificated Nurses – Class A*
(a) Women, who must be unmarried, or widows, are received for training in the Manchester Royal Infirmary, between the ages of 25 and 35.
They must be well educated; and they will be required to produce satisfactory references as to character, and a medical certificate of good health.

Personal application must be made to the Lady Superintendent of Nurses at the Hospital, between 10 and 12 a.m. No travelling expenses given.

(b) After a month's trial (for which period they do not receive wages or uniform) and on being approved, they will be expected to remain in the service of the Infirmary for three years. They will be subject to instant dismissal, however, at any time, in case of misconduct, or will be given a month's notice to leave if they should be considered inefficient, unsuitable, or are inattentive to their duties. During the period of training they will be employed in the Infirmary or at the Convalescent Hospital, Cheadle, as the Lady Superintendent may direct.

(c) They will be instructed in their duties by the 'Sisters' (Head Nurses), who will report every month to the Lady Superintendent as to the manner in which they perform their various duties; they will also receive Theoretical Instruction from members of the Honorary Staff of the Hospital, who deliver courses of Lectures to the Nurses on Medical and Surgical Nursing during each year.

(d) After the completion of three years' continuous service, and on being recommended by the Lady Superintendent of Nurses as having passed satisfactorily through the prescribed course of training and instruction, they will be examined in the months of January or July by a Committee of the Medical Board (if then in the employment of the Infirmary) and, if reported qualified, will be given certificates of efficiency and good conduct as Trained Nurses.

3. *Regulations affecting Certificated Nurses only – Class B*
(a) Certificated Nurses must give one calendar month's notice before leaving the service of the Hospital, and will receive the same from the Lady Superintendent; but, in case of misconduct, neglect of duty, or wilful disobedience, they will be liable to instant dismissal.

(b) Certificated Nurses may, if otherwise eligible, be promoted to the higher rank of 'Sister' (Head Nurse), to whom special rates of payment and a distinctive uniform are given and who are entitled to three weeks' holiday annually.

(c) Nurses of long and faithful service will be entitled to pensions.

4. *Regulations affecting both Certificated and Uncertificated Nurses*
(a) Uniform dress – consisting of 3 print dresses, 8 aprons, and 3 caps – is given to each uncertificated Nurse at the expiration of her month's trial, and to each certificated Nurse on engagement, and is renewed yearly. In the event of a Nurse leaving the Infirmary, from any cause, before the expiration of 12 months from date of last issue of her Uniform, its estimated value will be deducted from her wages. Nurses must wear their Uniform on all occasions when they are on duty. They must provide their own out-door dress, which should be plain and neat.

(b) All Nurses will be allowed seventeen days' leave of absence every year. They will also be given a day's holiday every month, provided the

Lady Superintendent can arrange for this without inconvenience to the work of the Hospital. Nurses must not absent themselves from the Hospital, nor from duty, without the permission of the Lady Superintendent.

(c) The Nurses are under the authority of the Lady Superintendent, who is responsible for the observance of these regulations.

(d) The following is the scale of payment, with board, laundry, and medical attendance, which will be given to uncertificated Nurses if engaged at the expiration of their month's trial and to certificated Nurses on engagement: 1st year, £10; 2nd year, £15; 3rd year, £18; 4th year, £20; after which the increase will be £1 annually up to a maximum of £25. Certificated Nurses employed on the Private Nursing Staff will receive, in addition to the above scale of wages, the sum of £5 per annum. Nurses on the Private Nursing Staff also receive one-half of the extra charge of 10s. 6d. per week made for each infectious or massage case nursed by them.

The Pensions remained the same.

There is a note in 1907 that £59 represented a quarter's wages for private nurses with £3 10s. for their travelling expenses.

On June 25, 1907, Miss Calvert resigned and the General Superintendent was instructed to advertise for a successor. It was reported that Sister Ellen G. Stephens, who had completed 34 years' service and who was now getting past working, proposed to retire on the pension of £25 per annum to which she was entitled under the terms of her engagement. The Medical Board recorded their high appreciation of the work done by Sister Stephens during the 34 years she had been on the Infirmary's staff and they expressed the regret which they feel at her departure.

She has worked loyally to carry out the aims of the Institution and her unostentatious faithful service has won the esteem of all who have been associated with her. She leaves behind many friends both among the staff and the patients who will never forget the kindly help she has given them in times past and who now wish her long continued health and every happiness in the rest she so well deserves.

In thanking Sister Stephens for her long period of service the Committee recorded that she had proved a capable and kindly nurse, devoted to her ward and her patients and loyal to those under whom she had served. They wished her every happiness in her retirement and hoped she would live many years to enjoy the pension she had earned by her long service.

One of Miss Calvert's last actions was to raise the question of the scale of pay of sisters, staff nurses, and private nurses. The General Superintendent was instructed to obtain particulars from other hospitals.

Miss Calvert was voted the sum of 100 guineas on her retirement at the end of the month, in recognition of her services during the 19 years (three at Monsall and sixteen at the Infirmary) she had been in the service of the Board of Management. (She did not qualify for a pension.) A week later she attended a meeting of the House Committee and was presented with the cheque. The minutes record:

During the whole of this long period Miss Calvert has deserved and possessed the absolute confidence of the Board and has carried out her duties to their entire satisfaction. She has displayed administrative abilities of quite a remarkable order, coupled with a kindly tactful control of her subordinates which has secured their loyal obedience and inspired their affectionate regard. The Board fully recognise that they are indebted to Miss Calvert's conspicuous ability and untiring energy for the high position the Manchester Royal Infirmary holds among the nurses' training schools in the country and they feel that her retirement is a serious loss to the Institution. Miss Calvert's uniform kindness and courtesy and her sympathetic assistance in times of stress and difficulty will be long remembered by all who have been associated with her in the work of the Infirmary and she will carry away with her their most cordial wishes for her health and happiness.

The Medical Board also passed a resolution:

The Medical Board desires to express its high appreciation of the long and faithful service of Miss F. Calvert, the Lady Superintendent, who for nearly twenty years has had charge of the nursing department of this Institution. The Board recognises the harmony which has characterised the working of the department during this period, has been due to Miss Calvert's excellent and judicious management. With respect to the education of the nurses, the staff, and especially those who have themselves acted as lecturers, thoroughly appreciate the large amount of time spent, the great pains taken and the ability and devotion displayed by Miss Calvert in this part of her work. The personal systematic education so faithfully given must now be bearing fruit in the after-efficiency of those who have passed through such a training. The staff would pay tribute not only to Miss Calvert's energy and capability but also to her uniform kindness and courtesy and those other qualities which lead beyond mere official recognition to friendship. They further desire to assure her that she will be long remembered in the Institution for her

F

excellent work and that she carries into her well-earned leisure the hearty appreciation and good wishes of those who have been associated with her in hospital life.

Although no portrait exists of Miss Calvert, there is a photograph of one of her nurses, Nurse Naden, who came from a medical family (Figure 6). She is seen standing in the large operating theatre at the old Infirmary. The students' gallery is in the background. The striking thing about her uniform is the ballooning shoulder sleeves. Sister Naden became theatre superintendent at the new Infirmary and remained in office well into the 1920's. It is thought the photograph was taken in 1902.

There is also the memory of a House Surgeon about two of the Sisters. 'Old Agnes' was a queer old thing in a large frilled cap standing at the surgeon's elbow in the theatre holding a skein of linen threads for ligatures in hands shaking from paralysis agitans. 'Old Mackin', the second surgical sister, was an enormous woman known as 'The Crimean Horse'. She had been one of Florence Nightingale's team of Sevastopol.

The new hospital was rapidly nearing completion. In little more than a year after Miss Calvert's departure the Old Infirmary would be empty.

It is important to realise that the work of the Infirmary was carried on by the Board of Management, which met quarterly or more often as necessary. The real work was done by the Infirmary Committee, which met weekly and was for many years known as the Weekly Board, whose minutes had to be ratified by the Board of Management, but as its important members served on the Infirmary Committee they were usually accepted without comment.

The minutes of the Medical Board went to the Infirmary Committee, where important points were discussed in detail and included in the Committee's minutes.

IO

Miss M. E. Sparshott, C.B.E., R.R.C.
1907-29

(a) Pre-War 1907-14

Miss Margaret Elwyn Sparshott was Matron of the Derbyshire Royal Infirmary at the time of her appointment. She had trained at Nottingham General Hospital where she had had the post of sister. Later she became night sister at Birmingham General Hospital and Matron at the District Hospital, Grimsby, before moving to Derby. She must have been 37 years of age at the time of her appointment.

She began by increasing the scale of pay for the certificated nursing staff which in 1908 was as follows: Sisters commence at £30 and rise by £2 a year to £40 p.a.; Staff Nurses commence at £22 and rise by £2 a year to £26 p.a.; Private Nurses commence at £28 and rise by £2 a year to £34 p.a. The maximum scale of pay had previously been £35, £25 and £30. It was also decided that Sisters should get four weeks' annual leave and all other nurses three weeks. Sisters had previously had three weeks and Nurses seventeen days.

Twenty-four extra nurses had been appointed in September 1908 because of the new hospital. They had to sleep there but were taken to the Old Infirmary in a special car.

There were further increases in salary scales: The Assistant Lady Superintendent and Home Sister £45, rising by £2 10s. to £55; the Night Superintendent £40, rising by £2 10s. to £50; Staff nurses performing theatre duties and in charge of Isolation, whose scale of pay was £22, rising by £2 to £26, were awarded a special duty allowance of £4 per annum.

The move from the Old Infirmary to the New took place on December 1, 1908. The work of transferring the patients to the new building was carried out with ease and smoothness that won the admiration of the patients themselves and said much for the care with which the whole business had been planned. The number of patients had been reduced to a minimum. Still there were few short of a hundred to be conveyed from the old building to the new and the work had to be done with every precaution in their interest. The raw December morning with fog hanging about the streets was not an ideal one for the purpose. There were five horse ambulances and Salford's new motor ambulance in use together with landaus and taxis, and the Infirmary's own omnibus that normally transported convalescent patients to Cheadle. The patients, warmly wrapped up, were carried down the hospital steps on chairs and stretchers and placed in the waiting vehicles. The journey took half-an-hour from bed to bed, and there were doctors, nurses and hot drinks to welcome them in their new wards. No patient complained of any discomfort. The majority relished a new experience and all were delighted at the 'new warm well-lighted wards with all the means of light and air and space that modern designs in the planning of hospitals have brought about'. The transfer started at noon and was completed within two hours. The last ambulance contained a number of students who drove away singing 'Auld Lang Syne'. One patient only was left. She was too ill to be disturbed. Apart from her room and the accident room the interior was deserted. The darkened windows and the big black dome brooded over a departed era.

The new building was formally opened by King Edward VII and Queen Alexandra on July 6, 1909. The ceremony took place in the out-patients' department and there the King knighted the Chairman of the Board of Management, William Cobbett.

Miss Sparshott proposed a new syllabus of lectures to the nursing staff:

	Lectures given by the Honorary Staff	Lectures given by the Nursing Staff
First-year nurses		
Nursing lectures		10 (by the Lady Superintendent)
Splint padding, Poultice making and Bandaging		16 (by the Assistant Lady Superintendent, Home Sister)
Second-year nurses		
Anatomy and physiology	10	
Ears	2	
Medical	10	
Gynæcology	4	
Dispensary	4	
Third-year nurses		
Surgery	10	
Ophthalmic	2	
Cookery		16
Massage		6
Total	**42**	**48**

The Lady Superintendent was authorised to carry out the programme in conjunction with certain members of the Honorary Staff. The increased expenditure from 30 to 42 guineas was approved. The syllabus was referred to the Medical Board but they did not think it went far enough. They felt that they should have been consulted about the details because so much nursing goes into the successful treatment of disease and because the Board teaches, examines and joins in certifying the competence of nurses, such a syllabus should be drawn up under their supervision and have their approval. They approved the outline of the syllabus but thought it required modification especially as regards the period of training at which it was proposed the subjects should be studied. For example, there should be instruction in elementary anatomy and physiology and hygiene in the first year of training. They wanted to be consulted in the production of a much more detailed syllabus.

As a further help to the education of Nurses, the Board decided to make a grant of £10 to the Nurses' Library plus an annual grant of £5 to be reconsidered if found insufficient.

The Board made a change to By-law 2 of the Lady Superintendent, making the rule read: 'She shall have the engagement, management and dismissal of all the Nurses over whom she is the responsible mistress, and such engagements and dismissals she shall immediately report to the General Superintendent *for transmission to the Infirmary Committee.*' The new words are in italics.

The certificate of Nurse Ross, who had burnt a patient with a hot water bottle, was withheld for six months.

War clouds were in the air as early as 1910. The Medical Department of the Royal Navy asked for sixteen nurses to be provided in war-time to supplement the staffs of the Naval Hospitals at Portsmouth, Plymouth and Chatham, and also possibly to proceed abroad or embark in hospital ships. The Infirmary authorities had already undertaken to provide a large number of nurses in connection with the Territorial scheme in war-time and could not provide others.

A Testimonial was granted to Miss Sparshott in 1910 in support of her application for the Matronship of St. Bartholomew's Hospital. But she was not appointed.

A detailed syllabus of instruction of Nurses was finally agreed upon. Forty-eight lectures were to be given by the Honorary Medical Staff and 46 by the Lady Superintendent and her staff. The syllabus was printed in detail.

The following scale of pay was adopted in 1910: Staff Nurses

£26 per annum; Private Nurses £30 per annum, rising £2 per annum and 5 per cent of the average earnings.

Miss Marie de Witt offered one hundred copies of her poems *The Passing of the King Belov'd* and *L'Entente Cordiale* to be sold by nurses at one shilling each for the benefit of the Hospital. This offer was declined with thanks.

Permission was granted to the Lady Superintendent of Nurses, as the Honorary Organising Matron of the 2nd Western General Hospital of the East Lancashire Territorial Force, to hold bed-making, bandaging and poultice-making lectures for ambulance men of the division.

Miss Sparshott's salary was increased in 1911 from £180 to £200 per annum.

There was a rearrangement of the heating pipes in the Nurses' Home so as to be able to heat the ground floor without heating the bedrooms.

The War Office asked if, in the event of war, a reserve of 25 nurses could be spared from the Infirmary staff. It was decided to start a scheme of registration of nurses completing their training who would be suitable and willing to serve. The War Office approved so the Lady Superintendent undertook to prepare the register.

The fees payable to the Infirmary for private nurses were increased: for ordinary medical and surgical cases from one-and-a-half to two guineas a week; for infectious and massage cases from two to two-and-a-half guineas a week.

Nurse Bourke, having scalded a patient, had her examination postponed for six months, and a notice was posted in the Nurses' dining-hall saying that in future any nurse who burned or scalded a patient from whatever cause would be dismissed.

It was decided in 1912 to convert a classroom in the Nurses' Home into a sitting-room for the Private Nurses.

In 1912 a ghost was seen in the nurses' home causing excitement amongst timid nurses and ward maids who pulled the sheets over their heads when they went to bed. It wasn't a white ghost with flowing drapery. Still less had it clanking chains and it certainly did not carry its head. It was a woman clad in a long black gown and stole, the only relief being its ghastly white face and long sinuous fingers and blanched, lifeless hands. It was seen first by a nurse who had come in late (we are not told what she had been doing that evening); seeing the figure ahead of her she thought it was a visitor gone astray so she hastened to show her the way. But as she raised her hand to touch her shoulder the woman vanished without a trace. When the story was told to her colleagues in the Home a search was made but nothing was found. Night porters and others lay in wait at strategic points. Their vigil was unavailing. But she still continued to haunt the Home. Ward maids saw the spectre disengage itself from curtains and dart across the passage in front of them to be swallowed up in a doorway or corridor or nothing. Pokers and flat-irons were finding their way into bedrooms but this did not deter the ghost. One young lady felt a clammy hand stretched over her face. 'Have you seen the lady in black?' became a catchword in the Home. At first it was thought the medical students were playing a joke but the investigations did not support that view. In the end it was decided that the ghost was the creation of an overwrought mind and gradually she ceased to appear, but not before many uncomfortable nights had been passed.

The Queen of Greece in 1913 wired asking if ten nurses could be supplied at once for the seat of war. This was the war between the Balkan States and Turkey. Eight members of the nursing staff volunteered, also two Infirmary trained nurses working at a Private Nursing Home. Suitable arrangements were made and it was reported a week later that they had arrived in Athens.

The scale of pay for Private Nurses was revised. This was increased to £40 per annum plus 5 per cent of the average fees.

Hospitals are always liable to damaging and untrue statements. A good example occurred in 1913. Miss Margaret Ashton gave an address on 'Woman's Realm' at a meeting of Women Liberals, at which she said:

> As an instance of how domestic affairs were mismanaged by men, when she visited the Royal Infirmary on one occasion she found that cotton blankets were being used whereas every workhouse infirmary in the country used woollen ones.

The Chairman, Sir William Cobbett, asked her if she had been correctly reported in the press. Miss Ashton replied in the affirmative, adding that she had spoken to her friend, Dr. Leech, about it. The Chairman thanked her for her letter, adding:

> The impression produced by your statement was that cotton blankets had recently been used at the Infirmary whereas Dr. Leech had died in July 1900. You must have been mistaken on that occasion of the visit

to which you refer for I am able to state, after most careful enquiry, that cotton blankets have never been used at the Infirmary.

There does not appear to have been a reply.

An historic adventure that caused much delight happened on New Year's Eve, 1913. It was customary to hold an annual dance on that night but strictly for nurses only. Men were rigidly excluded, although for many years residents and others had made more or less serious attempts to circumvent that regulation. Up to 1913 their efforts had proved futile.

The challenge was taken up by three residents – Freddy Bearn, C. H. Crawshaw, and Jackie Bennett. They hired costumes, Freddy going as a teddy-bear, the others as his keeper and a courtier dressed in blue, both masked (Figure 8). They sneaked into the dance hall through a side door and were astonished at some of the costumes they saw. Many of the nurses were dressed as men and many wore masks, which made things easier. They did not attempt to conceal their identity from the various partners with whom they danced and this ultimately proved their undoing. Things went very well, but there was a moment of panic when the Matron, who was sitting on a chair on a raised platform, called the bear over to her. Not knowing what to do he lay on his back in front of her, waving his paws in the air. She said, 'What a nice teddy-bear, who are you?' But he only growled.

More and more of the nurses heard what was going on and all eyes laughingly followed the trio. After about an hour and a half the nurse dancing with the bear whispered, 'They've spotted you.' She steered him to a door but it was locked, so she promptly fainted. Freddy picked her up and carried her to a bedroom and then with his colleagues he broke through the locked door and escaped. The costume was wrapped up and put under his bed. But it was clear next day that it had been undone and the secret was out.

The three were summoned before the Chairman but they sat with their mouths closed. He told them that they ought not to have gone to the dance and that they would be suspended for five days and would then have to appear before the Board. They had a most enjoyable holiday in the Lake District climbing Helvellyn and duly appeared before the Board on January 6. It is said that some of the members were secretly amused by the affair, but the General Superintendent, Mr. Carnt, was furious. He was much disliked by the residents and his temper had not been improved after an interview with the Resident Medical Officer, who had informed him that if the three were suspended any longer the rest of the residents would resign. This must be one of the earliest threats of hospital strike action. The situation was saved when the suggestion was made and accepted that they should write an apology to the Matron, and they were not even reprimanded. But Mr. Carnt relieved his feelings by writing this minute:

Special Board Meeting January 6, 1914
The General Superintendent reported to the Board that with the approval of the Chairman he had suspended three officers for breach of discipline in attending a private fancy-dress dance for the nurses on New Year's Eve in disguise and requested their appearance before the Board this morning.

It was resolved that if the officers apologised for their conduct they be severely reprimanded and restored to their duty.

The three officers concerned appeared before the Committee and expressed their deep regret for their conduct and undertook to sign an apology to the Lady Superintendent of Nurses and the Nursing Staff.

The Chairman administered a severe reprimand and informed them that the Committee had decided to accept their apology and to restore them to duty.

The adventure remained a delightful talking point for many years. It had an amusing sequel. When the 1914 war broke out Dr. Bearn enlisted and when he left the hospital a probationer presented him with a small teddy-bear mascot. It lost one eye in an early battle and its second eye on the Somme, and it won its owner the D.S.O. and the Military Cross. When the war broke out again its eyes were replaced and it was taken once more to France. It was evacuated safely with Dr. Bearn through Dunkirk after much anxiety.

War was getting nearer. The Hospital authorities were asked by the Red Cross Society if they could train their nurses for periods of three months in the wards. But as there was no residential accommodation available it was suggested and accepted that six nurses should have three months' training in the casualty and out-patients' departments provided they attended diligently and wore the Red Cross uniform.

The Greek Minister sent a letter enclosing medals and diplomas conferred by the Queen Mother of Greece upon Miss Davidson, Miss Gooseman, Miss Cowie, Miss Sloan, Miss Jackson, Miss Gordon, Miss Green, Miss Scott and Miss Mason, who had served with distinction as nurses in Greece during the war. The Chairman undertook to make the presentations and the nurses were photographed with Miss Sparshott outside the main entrance of the hospital.

The year 1914 saw the inauguration of a local branch of the National Union of Trained Nurses. The movement had started in a little town in Somerset fifteen years earlier and by now, with London as its centre, there were twenty-eight branches in local and provincial towns. The Union aimed at fostering a sense of comradeship and maintaining the highest ideals in this branch of social service. I cannot find any reference in the literature to this Union; possibly it was the National Council of Nurses, which consisted of qualified nurses and had been founded by Mrs. Gordon Fenwick.

There were a few changes in the new Regulations for the engagement of nurses from those of 1906, but uncertificated nurses desiring training had to be between 23 and 30 years of age (previously 25 to 35). No testimonial would be given to uncertificated nurses but prospective employees could refer to the Lady Superintendent. Leave of absence for all nurses was increased from seventeen to twenty-one days a year. The scale of pay was unchanged except for nurses who became certificated and were retained as staff nurses. Their pay would be £26 per annum. Certificated nurses employed on the private nursing staff would receive £40 per annum plus 5 per cent of the average annual fees, also one-half of the extra charge of 10s. 6d. per week made for each infectious or massage case nursed by them, and out-door as well as in-door uniforms. This was a considerable increase. The scale of pensions was unchanged.

And so we reach World War I and an immense burden of extra work for Miss Sparshott and her nurses.

(b) The War Years 1914-18

Miss Sparshott's administrative ability and the energy and skill of her nursing staff were stretched to the utmost during the war years. Early in October 1914, 250 beds were provided for military patients and were immediately occupied by wounded soldiers. The accommodation was extended as necessity arose until 520 out of a total of 884 beds were reserved for military cases. (In peace-time and with two extra wards the number of beds available nowadays numbers 676. But they are rarely all available.)

As early as the end of 1914 the Committee placed on record its appreciation of the cheerful and willing manner in which the staff of the hospital of all ranks had carried out the considerable amount of extra duty caused by the establishment of 208 additional beds for military patients and the consequent reception and treatment of a great number of additional patients. Little did they know what was to come. M3, 4 and 5 units housed medical cases. The day rooms on M4 and M5 housed surgical cases. These were also treated in the large male wards and day rooms on S1, 3 and 5. Ear cases were treated in the aural wards. There were twenty-four beds in the teaching block, which was otherwise entirely occupied by students and residents. The X-ray department was not there until the early 20's. Officers were treated in the side wards on S4, and there was a full-scale hospital in the Central Branch. The reception of soldiers continued until the early summer of 1919 and the last of these patients was transferred to various military disposal hospitals in August. During this period 10,077 soldiers were admitted; 8,197 surgical and 1,880 medical cases. The operations performed numbered 3,958. With a depleted nursing staff, which at one time dropped to 190, the Infirmary had established within its walls a military hospital of considerable dimensions.

Miss Sparshott had other duties for she was Principal Matron of the military hospital in Whitworth Street, known as the 2nd Western General Hospital, which became the base of twenty-two auxiliary hospitals in Manchester, Salford and Stockport all working in unison under the guidance of Miss Sparshott. There were 3,800 beds and 630 Sisters and Nurses at the disposal of the military authorities. Many of them had been trained in the wards of the Infirmary, and all the time she was sending nurses to Army and Naval hospitals at home and abroad. The Royal recognition of her work, first with the Royal Red Cross, and at the end of the war the C.B.E. was richly earned.

The Matron at Whitworth Street, Miss Woodhouse, an Infirmary-trained nurse, also received the R.R.C., and more than fifty sisters and nurses trained at the Infirmary received the associate R.R.C. Several were mentioned in despatches and Sister Sloane was presented by the President of the French Republic with a medal in silver gilt. While all this was going on the minutes record other happenings.

In April 1915 a war bonus of £10 was granted to certified nurses who remained for twelve months after January 1, 1915, or after the date of their certificate if it was later. This was to have repercussions four years later.

Permission was granted to place four bronze memorial plates in the Chapel in memory of Nurses Johnson, Modsley, Stone and Begbie who had died in the service of the institution. Later in the year Sister French, in charge of S1M died after only two days' illness. She had given 33 years of loyal and devoted service to the hospital and the Committee recorded their appreciation in the minutes. The sum of £70 was soon collected for a memorial, and an anonymous donor promised £50 more if the memorial took the form of a stained glass window in the chapel. This idea was accepted and in due course the window was unveiled at a Service of Dedication conducted by the Lord Bishop of Manchester.

The Chairman reported in 1916 that of the twenty-seven nurses who obtained their certificate, four had been permanently retained on the staff, four temporarily for holiday duty, at the usual rate for Sisters – £30 per annum, and a bonus of £10 at the conclusion of every twelve months' service during the war. The remainder were asked what terms would satisfy them. They asked for £40 per annum plus a £10 bonus but were not retained on those terms. The salaries of the Assistant Matron (Miss Mundy), the Home Sister (Miss Smith), and the Matron-in-Charge of Central Branch were increased in 1916 to £80 per annum.

Up to now there has been no mention that I can find that the Lady Superintendent took any part in the final examination of the nurses although I always imagined that she did, but in July 1916 Miss Sparshott asked the Medical Board if they would agree to an invitation being sent to a Lady Superintendent from another hospital to co-operate with her in an honorary capacity.

Sixteen junior Sisters asked for an increase in their salary from £30 to £40 per annum in 1916. It was pointed out that with the addition of the £10 war bonus their position was in line with the junior Sisters at other hospitals. They hadn't long to wait however. In order to compare favourably with other institutions the following salary changes were made in 1917:

Sisters and certified nurses commence at £42 rising by £5 in two years to £52. Probationers : £12 in their first year, £17 in their second and £22 in their third year. Members of the nursing staff would be pensioned at £52 p.a. after 25 years' service as a certified nurse. Any nurse who had attained the age of 50, had served the hospital continuously for not less than 25 years, and being unfit for further work and of satisfactory character would receive a pension of £25 per annum payable quarterly as long as they behaved themselves.

On the same day it was decided to purchase a piano for the Nurses' Home at the cost of £41 8s.

A shocking thing happened in August 1917. Three nurses purchased some champagne, conveyed it to the Infirmary and consumed it in Nurse H.'s bedroom. After consideration of the circumstances the Board resolved that two of the nurses be dismissed forthwith and that Nurse H. be severely reprimanded and her examination be postponed until June 1918.

During the same year Queen Mary visited certain wards occupied by soldiers. She was very pleased with what she saw and with the arrangements that had been made for her visit.

As was the case after the second world war there was time to think of big national problems. In 1915 the Hon. Arthur Stanley, M.V.O., M.P., Chairman of the Joint War Committee of the British Red Cross Society, asked the Board to approve the broad outlines of a scheme having as its object the co-operation of training schools for nurses and the institution of a College of Nursing with its Council of Management and Examination Board. The Committee approved, but in view of present circumstances thought the matter should be deferred.

Miss Sparshott now took a hand in things. Six months later she approached the Chairman of the Board (Sir William Cobbett) and they wrote to the Hon. Arthur Stanley suggesting that a meeting should be arranged at the Infirmary. It took place on July 28, 1916, in the Out-Patients' Department. Six hundred people attended. A Bill was to be presented to Parliament to promote the foundation of the College.

But the Board were not happy with the articles of association of the College. They were unanimous in thinking the proposed constitution of the Council of the College raised a grave objection to the scheme. They considered that while nurses should be represented on the Council, medical and laymen ought also to be included, all three classes in equal proportions, and that unless a rearrangement of the scheme on this or some similar basis could be adopted the feeling of the Board was that they could not continue to give the scheme their support. The Hon. Arthur Stanley pointed out that the constitution of the Council had been left blank for the time being. He asked the Board to suspend their judgment of the Bill until they saw it in its final form. When they did so they must have had a profound shock.

At this stage we should look at the story of the foundation of the college at national level. There had been, from 1887 when it was founded by Mrs. Gordon Fenwick, a Royal British Nurses' Association. With a progressive outlook, it aimed at improving education and training, and worked indefatigably for State Registration. But it did not get very far mainly because the British Medical Association would not support State Registration. In 1902 a Society for the State Registration of Nurses was formed and a series of unsuccessful Bills were introduced into Parliament. A Select Committee of the House of Commons was appointed to consider the question, and although it was in sympathy with the project, nothing tangible resulted and nothing had been done when the war broke out.

The war raised problems that had not hitherto faced the nursing profession. The care of the wounded called for a very high standard of knowledge and nursing skill. Early in 1916 some leaders of the profession under the guidance of Dame Sarah Swift and Sir Arthur Stanley (the Matron-in-Chief and Chairman of the British Red Cross Society) together with the Medical Superintendent of Guy's Hospital met to discuss the possibilities of forming an organisation that would be self-governing and which would assist and direct nurses in all stages of their professional life. They drafted the Constitution of the College of Nursing on simple democratic lines and it was registered in March 1916 under the Companies Act of 1908–13 as a company limited by guarantee and not having a share capital. There had been hot opposition by the Royal British Nurses' Association but in the end they joined the College.

The first object of the College was to set a definite uniform standard for membership and also for nursing training to be adopted by English hospitals, for this was before the advent of State Registration. I am indebted to the secretary of the Royal College of Nursing for the following information:

In January, 1916, the Hon. Arthur Stanley suggested that the promoters of the College of Nursing should appoint the first Council of Management, two-thirds of whom should be matrons of hospitals or superintendents of nursing. In subsequent discussions there were objections to this proposal because it was felt that nurses would only be represented on the Council through their matrons. Others objected to laymen on the Council. Miss Haughton who was a member of the Council stated in March, 1916, that 'two-thirds, at least, of the Council of Management shall be matrons of hospitals or superintendents of nursing, or sisters and nurses still engaged in the active practice of their profession, the remaining members being medical men or women and men or women of administrative experience to help on the business side of the undertaking. The number of members of Council shall not be less than fifteen nor more than thirty (unless determined by a general meeting). When the College has been established, vacancies on the Council will be filled from year to year by the votes of the members'.

The first meeting of the Council of the College of Nursing Ltd., was held on April 1, 1916, at 83 Pall Mall (The Royal Automobile Club) which was also its first registered office. The membership of the Council as appointed by the signatories to the articles of association was: Miss R. Cox-Davies, R.R.C., Matron, Royal Free Hospital; Miss A. Lloyd Still, C.B.E., R.R.C., Matron, St. Thomas's Hospital; Miss S. A. Swift, R.R.C., Matron-in-Chief, Joint War Committee, British Red Cross Society and Order of St. John of Jerusalem; Miss J. Melrose, R.R.C., Matron, Royal Infirmary, Glasgow; Miss A. Hughes, late General Inspector, Q.V.J.N.I. Nurses; Miss Jane Walker, M.D.; Miss L. V. Haughton, Matron, Guy's Hospital; Miss M. E. Ray, R.R.C., Matron, King's College Hospital; Miss A. W. Gill, R.R.C., Lady Superintendent, Royal Infirmary, Edinburgh; Miss A. B. Baillie, R.R.C., Matron, Royal Infirmary, Bristol; Miss M. E. Sparshott, R.R.C., Lady Superintendent, Royal Infirmary, Manchester; The Hon. Arthur Stanley, M.P., M.V.O.; Sir Cooper Perry, M.D., F.R.C.P.; Mr. Comyns Berkeley, M.C., M.A., M.D., F.R.C.P. (later Hon. Treasurer); Dr. H. G. Turney, F.R.C.P.; Col. James Cantlie, F.R.C.S.; Miss A. C. Gibson, Matron, The Infirmary, Birmingham; Mr. W. Minet, Governor of St. Thomas's Hospital. The first Council was appointed but, from 1918 onward, one-third of the members thereof retired. Elections to the Council were held in 1918-1919-1920 so that the first fully-elected Council took office in 1920.

The Hon. Arthur Stanley was elected Chairman and Sir Cooper Perry temporary Hon. Secretary. The Council co-opted the following extra members: Miss E. Barton, R.R.C., Matron, Chelsea Infirmary; Prof. J. Glaister, M.D., University of Glasgow; Miss A. McIntosh, C.B.E., R.R.C., Matron, St. Bartholomew's Hospital; Miss E. Mowat, Matron, Whitechapel Infirmary; Miss E. M. Musson, R.R.C., Matron, Birmingham General Hospital; Miss C. E. Vincent, R.R.C., Lady Superintendent, Royal Infirmary, Leicester; Miss Seymour Yapp, Superintendent Nurse, Ashton-under-Lyne Infirmary. The twenty-five strong council was made up therefore of: sixteen Matrons, one Superintendent Nurse, five Medical men, one Medical woman and two laymen.

Thought was already being given in 1917 to the building of a new nurses' home but land had to be acquired. In September 1917 Sir William Cobbett was given permission to purchase Nos. 1 and 23 York Place at any price up to £2,200. He bought them for £2,225 and there had to be a further payment of £225. The Board approved.

The College having been successfully launched, Miss Sparshott presided in June 1918 over a meeting of eighty Matrons, all members of the College, to discuss the State Registration of nurses. Her salary must have been increased for we find her expressing thanks to the Board for their appreciation of her work, also for the increase in her salary.

Further progress was made when the Board asked the Medical Board to appoint two external examiners for nurses, one physician and one surgeon, to act in conjunction with two internal examiners, the external examiners to be paid an honorarium of three guineas provided they resided in the locality of the Infirmary. In July 1921 the pass list was signed for the first time by the examiners including E. Maud Smith, M. E. Sparshott, and R. W. Marsden, who was Medical Superintendent of Crumpsall Hospital.

Sister Reid retired in 1918. She was awarded the full retirement pension of £52 per annum for her long and faithful service extending over 35 years. It will be seen shortly that this wasn't enough. She became something of a legend for very many years. Dr. A. T. Wilkinson was especially renowned as a diagnostician in the days when powers of observation and clinical experience were all that were available. On his ward rounds he would often ask Sister Reid for her opinion and once there was a classical reply: 'Sister, do you think this is a case of new growth or an aneurysm?' To which she replied: 'He has his bowels moved like an aneurysm,' and she was right.

The pension granted to Sister Arthur was increased from £35 to £52 per annum. Woollen jerseys were provided for the night nurses at an approximate cost of £50.

The year 1918 ended with a catastrophic national epidemic of influenza. Visitors to patients were stopped except for those on the free list. But the way in which it struck the nursing staff is a matter for the next section but one. It is time to learn Miss Sparshott's views on the nursing profession.

(c) Miss Sparshott's Views on the Profession of Nursing

Nursing was, until the Dissolution of the Monasteries, carried out by the religious. After this, nursing was done by women of no education and often poor character. The ridicule by Dickens in *Martin Chuzzlewit* in 1843 stirred the conscience of many as to the conditions in our hospitals, and amongst those roused were Florence Nightingale, Elizabeth Fry, and Agnes Jones.

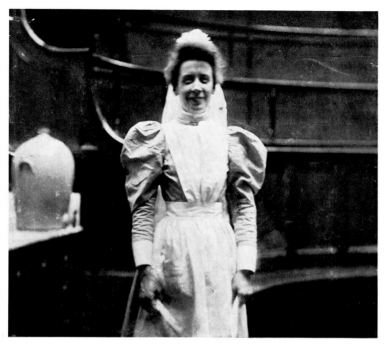

6 Theatre Nurse Naden, 1902

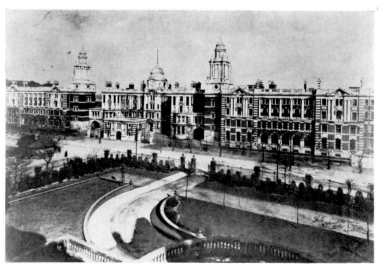

7 M.R.I. 1910

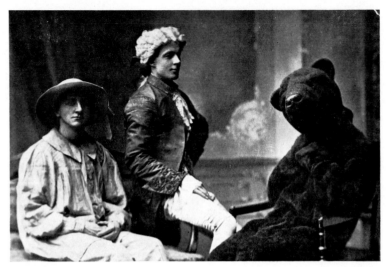

8 The three housemen who gatecrashed the nurses' fancy dress dance

THE GENERAL REGISTER OF NURSES.

Reg. No.	Name (if Married, Maiden Name)	Permanent Address	Date of Registration	Qualifications
1	Fenwick (née Manson) Ethel Gordon	20, Upper Wimpole St London. W1.	30.9.1921	Royal Infirmary Manchester. Trained 1878 - 1879
2	Still Alicia Frances Jane Lloyd	S. Thomas' Hosp. S.E.1.	30.9.1921	S. Thomas' Hospital London Trained 1896 - 1899
3	Cox-Davies Rachel	2 Grenville Street, Brunswick Square, London W.C.1. Royal Free Hospital	30.9.1921	S. Bartholomew's Hospital

9 The first nurses' register

When Florence Nightingale returned from the Crimean War the nation gave her £70,000, and with this money she started the first modern training school of nurses at the Hospital of St. Thomas (founded 1213), and now the Nightingale School of Nurses is renowned throughout the world. As time has gone on, and with it the advance of medicine and surgery, the need for nurses has steadily increased.

About the only profession for women not overstocked is that of nursing. Many helpers are wanted in our hospitals and nursing homes, and in the Public Health Services as District Nurses, Welfare Workers, Health Visitors, and School Nurses. There is a great demand for nurses in the Navy, Army, Air Force, and Prison Services, and in many of our Colonies; the call also comes from the Foreign Mission Field. There is no end to the possibilities for the woman who takes up nursing.

The nurse is the one who is allowed to see patients at their weakest moments, to tend friends in their darkest hours, to bring unseen strength by giving of her own strength. The avenues by which a nurse may help are untold, and the responsibilities are correspondingly great. No one should think of taking up nursing who has not the mother instinct strongly developed. One of the reasons why more girls do not take up this work is because in our modern life that instinct is rather in the background at the present time.

To my mind there is no grander life for a young woman. The training days are hard, but not harder than many others; the work is difficult and at first trying; but the three years of training pass all too soon, having been lived in happy community life, where life-long friends are often made. The practical work itself, in the early days, is tedious to some, but gradually this work, which is essential if we are hoping in the future to teach others, passes.

The study, to the girl with only elementary education, is hard, but by no means impossible. As in any other profession, the more educated the girl, the better are her chances of future advancement. The girl is not left to struggle alone in her studies, as is thought by some. Doctors, matrons, and ward sisters have been and are teachers, and latterly a trained nurse, with special qualifications as tutor, has been added to the staff of all large hospitals.

No premium is required for training, but a small sum is supplied as pocket money. In addition, free board, lodging, laundry, and part uniform are supplied. Doctor's attendance and nursing care in illness are provided.

When the training days are over the nurse can then decide what branch of nursing she will prefer to take up, and whether she will remain in her own country or try life further afield. It would be difficult to find another profession which embraces all types of women, with the scope to develop their powers along the lines they feel themselves best fitted for. The essential qualifications are good health, the desire to live for

G

others, perseverance, patience, cheerfulness, adaptability, and common sense. Given these qualifications, the life of usefulness in the service of humanity and in humble dependence on the Father of all must be a happy life.

(d) 1919-28

The influenza epidemic was almost a national disaster. Whole wards were filled with patients and there were very many deaths from a cyanotic pneumonia. One ward on M5 was filled with sick nurses and there were at one time 55 suffering from the disease. There were at least two deaths and once a state of near panic.

Much of the trouble was due to the after effects of the war, in particular, tight rationing of food, and, as far as the nurses were concerned, they were grossly overworked. There was a letter in the *Manchester Guardian* on the point:

> Being until a few days ago a patient in the Manchester Royal Infirmary I was astonished to learn the long hours that the nurses put in – both day and night nurses. They are expected to be always cheerful and on the alert to perform all kinds of work. The great majority of them take up this profession because of a great love of humanity and therefore go about their arduous tasks and endure these long hours on that account. I think it is the duty of the community to see to it that the hours and conditions of this indispensable section of the workers are made shorter and brighter and brought more into line with other professions.

Unfortunately nothing could be done about it. There was no room for more nurses. What was needed was a new nurses' home. But there was a small relief. The attendance of the nursing staff at evening prayers was no longer compulsory. A by-law had to be rescinded.

The first resident Sister Tutor to the Nursing Staff was appointed in 1919 at a salary of £100 per annum. Miss Abram had previously been in charge of S3M. The hospital may have been a bit slow here, for the first Sister Tutor of all had been appointed at St. Thomas's Hospital several years previously. But probably the war was responsible for the delay.

The College was expanding fast. One small room for a headquarters office was no longer sufficient. By 1919 it was necessary to rent a whole house. Three years later it had a home of its own and a Royal Patron in the late Queen Mary. Finally, in 1928, it was incorporated by Royal Charter and became the Royal College of Nursing – the word 'limited' could at last be dropped.

State Registration became law in December 1919, the basis of the Bill having largely been drafted by the College. This Nurses' Registration Act, which is the basic control of the profession today, marked the end of Mrs. Gordon Fenwick's long campaign. It was right and proper that her name should be put first on the Register together (Figure 9) with the statement that she had trained at the Manchester Royal Infirmary 1878–79. Actually there were three acts, one for England and Wales, one for Scotland and one for Ireland. Each country was empowered to set up a General Nursing Council, to compile a recommended syllabus of instruction and a compulsory syllabus for examination, and to organise qualifying examinations throughout the country. The Council was also authorised to compile and maintain a Register of duly qualified nurses and of satisfactory nurses already in practice.

Back at home there was a complaint about the nurses' suppers. The Chairman inspected the meal on two occasions and found them 'satisfactory in most respects. Wherever the fare appeared meagre it would be increased and varied as opportunity permitted'. The Sisters asked that their evening meal should be apart from the nurses, an alternative dish when cheese or tripe or curry or macaroni were served and better food generally; also the fulfilment of the promise of an annual war bonus so long as the war lasted. This promise had not been fulfilled since the end of 1916. The Board undertook to try to implement the first, would try to improve the food, but rationing still made things difficult. The third point was founded on a misapprehension – the war bonus had been found to work unfairly, therefore an increased wage of £1 a month (£12 a year) was substituted and has been paid ever since December 1916.

For a short time facilities for rest and convalescence were provided. Mr. and Mrs. Tatton offered accommodation at Cuerdon Hall, and during the eighteen months before the Board found it necessary to close the arrangement 243 Sisters and Nurses had benefited from a stay there. The Board were grateful and presented Miss Murray, the Matron, with eight guineas in recognition of the attention and consideration shown by her.

It was only just that the period of service in the Army or Navy of any member of the nursing staff during the war should be considered as service to the Infirmary so far as seniority, increase of salary and pension were concerned.

G*

The nursing staff in 1920 consisted of the Lady Superintendent, the Assistant Lady Superintendent, one Home Sister, one Sister Tutor, Two Night Sisters, twenty-two Ward Sisters, thirteen Certificated Nurses and 200 Probationers, giving a total of 241. There were also one Matron, one Night Sister and two Ward Sisters at the Convalescent Hospital, Cheadle, and one Sister-in-Charge, one Night Sister and one Day Sister at the Central Branch. But these were not sufficient. A Committee was appointed in 1920 and produced a report containing the following extracts, beginning with Miss Sparshott's Report:

I beg to report that I am finding difficulty in obtaining probationers. During my absence from duty I have visited several Hospitals, and compared notes with various Matrons, and we are all experiencing the same difficulty. The chief reasons for the scarcity are: (1) There are so many more branches of work open to women. (2) The foolish and untrue statements regarding nursing work which have appeared in the lay press. (3) The fact that women can enter many occupations at an earlier age. (4) The long hours of work, and the comparatively small remuneration after the Certificate is gained.

I have only, for a short period, been able to keep my numbers of probationers up to the 230 sanctioned, and for which we have bed accommodation including the 25 beds in Lister House. Since March of this year my numbers have never been above 210 and are now down to 201. I have four names of probationers waiting to come in on October 1, and four of the staff are leaving. You know the great rush of work in this Infirmary, and this, for the nurses, is made much heavier by the fact that servants and charwomen are most difficult to obtain. I have been able to give annual holidays correctly, and the usual daily leave in most cases; but I beg to point out that our day nurses work 68 hours a week, and night nurses 77 hours. We shall not get more probationers until we can reduce the hours of work.

May I suggest:

1. *That two Units be closed,* thus releasing 28 nurses (17 Surgical, 11 Medical); by this means I shall be able to reduce the hours of work.

2. *Take probationers at the age of* 19 instead of 21 (girls are allowed to enter the Medical Profession at 18).

3. *Start a Preliminary Training School;* this would mean that for the first two months the probationer would work entirely under the Sister Tutor, and pass an examination before entering the Wards. This will give the younger girl an easier moral and physical entrance to the Wards and ensure that a certain standard is reached.

4. *Advertise* our advantages both in the Lay and Nursing Press.

Other Hospitals are offering the following inducements; they are making a fourth year of training, and during that year teach their better Nurses – Midwifery, Massage or Housekeeping. This, at present, I do not wish to recommend, as I feel the poorer type of Nurse only would be available for work in the Wards, and no benefit would accrue to the Infirmary.

I append a comparision of Salaries between ourselves and the Withington Hospital – these are often quoted by my staff:

	M.R.I.	Withington	
		Salary	Bonus
Sisters	£65 by £5 to £75	£55 by £5 to £75	+33⅓%
Staff Nurses	£50 by £5 to £60	£45 by £2 10s. to £60	+33⅓%
Probationers			
3rd year	£30	£30	+33⅓%
2nd year	£22	£26	+33⅓%
1st year	£18	£22	+33⅓%
Dining Hall Maids	£19 – £28	£22 – £2 – £28	+£29 14s.*
House Maids	£19 – £30	£18 – £2 – £24	+£24 6s.*

* Based on Civil Service Bonuses

Reference Suggestion 1. The present 77-hour week for Night Nurses can be reduced to a 56-hour week by giving two hours off each night, and two nights a fortnight; 17 additional nurses will be required if one Medical and one Surgical Unit is closed. The closing of one Medical and one Surgical Unit will release 28 Nurses, of whom 17 would be employed on night duty as above. The other 11 would be used to fill in the vacancies on day duty, so that the Nurses will get their day off a month, but no reduction of their present 68-hour week until the existing 30 vacancies on the staff are filled. Their hours can then be reduced somewhat, but not to 56.

The Committee reported as follows:

The number of Nurses required in order to reduce the working hours to the standard generally adopted and recommended, is 295. As accommodation has not hitherto been provided at the Infirmary for that number, the Lady Superintendent has been authorised to employ 230. She has been unable to obtain this number, and there are now 201 only, and so far it has been found impossible to increase the number. In order to do so, it is necessary to make the occupation more attractive. A cardinal requisite for this purpose is to reduce the number of working hours. These at present are for Day Nurses 68 and for Night Nurses 77 hours per week, and it is desirable to reduce them to 56. This can be done in the case of Night Nurses by closing 2 Units, 1 Medical (50 beds) and

1 Surgical (60 beds), which will release 28 Nurses (11 Medical and 17 Surgical) of whom 17 will be employed on Night Duty. The remaining 11 will be used to make good the deficiency in the Day Staff.

It is with the greatest reluctance that the Sub-Committee recommend the closing of the two Units, and the Medical Member of the Sub-Committee is strongly opposed to it, and voted against it. The Committee is however, unable to suggest any other effective alternative, and recommend that it should be done.

With reference to suggestions 2, 3 and 4 of the report, the Committee are unanimously in favour of adopting them subject as regards number 3 that it is practicable to adapt two of the houses in York Place as a Home for 15 Probationer Nurses.

The Committee unanimously recommend that By-laws Section 9 on Page 50, Section 19 on page 57, and Section 6 on page 59, be rescinded, and that their place be taken by the following:—

> The Staff shall attend Divine Service, when this can be arranged without inconvenience to the work of the Hospital, at 9-30 a.m. on Sunday – all other Chapel Services are optional.

W. Cobbett,

October 8, 1920.   Chairman.

When the report was considered by the Board of Management, recommendations 2, 3 and 4 were adopted. Recommendation 1 (the closure of wards) was postponed.

It was vital to make immediate plans for the erection of a Nurses' Home in York Place. The hospital owned No. 1 York Place, which housed massage students, and the two vacant houses Nos. 13 and 15. Immediate notice to quit was given to the tenants of houses Nos. 3, 21 and 23 and the Corporation was asked for permission to demolish houses 1, 3, 21 and 23 and to enclose on the north side of York Place with a road surrounding the island site.

Mr. and Mrs. R. P. Goldschmidt 'presented the valuable and acceptable gift of a pianoforte' to the Nurses' Home. Next year a piano was purchased for the Nursing Staff at the Central Branch.

A deputy Home Sister was appointed in 1921 and permission was given to Miss Sparshott to entertain for a fortnight annually two international student nurses who were interested in English hospitals and wanted an insight into the methods of nursing in this country. She was also provided with a spare bedroom, the Board taking advantage of the discontinuation of a resident medical post.

There was still great concern about the shortage of Nurses. Miss Sparshott was asked to produce a report on the engagement of Probationers.

Report from the Lady Superintendent of Nurses re the engagement of Probationers

On receiving an enquiry, unless the letter asking for forms is either untidy or illiterate, the forms are sent, with the request that they are returned filled in, in applicant's own handwriting with a letter stating how she has been engaged during the last five years. On the return of the form, if the letter shows signs of ability to write decently and with good composition, references are asked for from the persons named as referees on the form. If these references are satisfactory, the applicant is asked to come for an interview, if they are unsatisfactory, the applicant receives a letter stating that she is not one selected.

As far as possible, I like to have girls with Secondary School Education or education in an Elementary School with further tuition as a minimum. We find that girls who have had no School Education since the age of 13 or 14 are incapable of taking advantage of the Lectures and Tuition provided for them here: and, also, they come (as a rule) from homes where they have not had the Home Education which is necessary for them to sit at meals and mix socially with our other probationers, or to take their place as useful nurses capable of fitting in to any position they may be called on to fill later.

I am glad to be able to report that since our salaries have been raised, we are receiving more applicants of a suitable type, and that by April 1 I shall have my full staff of 230 nurses, and, also, have a waiting list for any probable vacancies which may occur. I shall, therefore, be able to continue nursing the present wards without curtailment of beds, but of course, without the reduction of nurses' hours which is so necessary.

(Signed) *M. E. Sparshott.*

February 17, 1921.

The salary of seven senior Sisters was increased by £15 a year and the pension given to Sister Reid was raised to £78 per annum, the Board being informed that she was in some financial difficulty. The first reunion of Nurses took place in 1921. Sir William Milligan suggested that there should be more relaxation for Nurses. This was essential. He thought that, if approached, the Corporation Baths Committee might make special arrangements for the Nurses to use the near-by swimming bath. This seems to have happened for an active swimming club was organised.

An alteration was made to By-law 2 concerning the Lady Superintendent. The full By-laws now read as follows, the additional part being in italics.

XXX – *Lady Superintendent of Nurses*

1. She shall be a fully trained nurse, possessing a certificate of not less than three years' training, and shall not be less than 30 nor more than 40 years of age on appointment.

2. She shall reside in the hospital, and devote the whole of her time to the performance of her duties. *Any intended absence* for a day or a night shall *be notified by her in advance* to the general superintendent.

3. She shall have the engagement, management, and dismissal of all the nurses, over whom she is the responsible mistress, and such engagements and dismissals she shall immediately report to the general superintendent, for transmission to the Infirmary Committee. She shall report to the general superintendent, for transmission to the Infirmary Committee if desirable, any circumstances of difficulty or irregularity connected with her department.

4. She shall visit alternately half the wards every day, the remaining half being visited by the assistant lady superintendent on her behalf, and shall ascertain, from personal observation when necessary, that the duties of the night nurses are efficiently performed.

5. She shall see that the wards, offices, beds, linen, and everything within her department are kept clean and in good order.

6. She shall prepare once a year an inventory of the beds, bedding, linen, etc., in use in the wards, and forward the same to the general superintendent.

7. In case the diets be not efficiently prepared and punctually received, she shall report the same to the general superintendent.

8. She shall enter in a book to be provided for the purpose all particulars relating to the employment of nurses in private families, and shall make all arrangements and conduct the correspondence relating thereto. She shall prepare a list, once in each quarter, of all the nurses, ward, hall, and home maids under her control, with their respective salaries, and forward the same to the general superintendent, for transmission to the Infirmary Committee.

9. She shall attend, with all the nurses who can be spared from their duties, and who have no conscientious objections, evening prayers at the times appointed. She shall see that the nurses and the ward, hall, and home maids, as far as practicable, attend divine service on Sundays, either at the chapel of the Infirmary or at some other place of worship.

10. She shall give a course of instruction to the nurses annually, and be responsible for their general training.

11. She shall hold her office subject to a three months' notice, in writing, from or to the Board.

Outside sleeping accommodation was still a problem. On one occasion in 1921 an advertisement was published in *The Evening News:*

Sleeping Accommodation (only)
Required for Lady Nurses: vicinity of High Street, Chorlton-on-Medlock : quote terms and details of accommodation offered – V.2. E.N.

There were 32 replies. Beds offered numbered 52, 22 of which were unsuitable! The Committee decided it was not advisable to have Infirmary nurses housed in this manner.

A meeting of the College of Nursing was held in the Out-Patients' Department. Thereafter the East Lancashire Branch was given permission to hold regular meetings in the Infirmary.

Miss Sparshott became seriously ill in 1922 and was off work for four-and-a-half months. But she was 'completely restored to health' when she returned to duty.

A disarticulated skeleton and a set of anatomical charts were purchased for £25 for the teaching of nurses.

The Board of Management announced in August 1922 that £100,000 was wanted to build a nurses' home and that the nursing staff were going to hold a three-day bazaar in November to raise funds for this purpose. There had been a great expansion of the hospital's work since the new building had been opened in 1908 with accommodation for 189 nurses. Increase in staff meant that many nurses had to be lodged outside. This was an inconvenience. Nurses on night duty worked a 73-hour week and those on day duty did a 63-hour week. It was agreed that these hours were much too long. The Board were anxious to reduce duty hours for all nurses to 56 hours, which would mean that 65 more nurses would be required. It was to accommodate these and bring all the nurses under one roof that the new home was required.

The Bazaar was opened by Viscountess Cowdray on the Wednesday, Lady Donner on the Thursday and the singer, Miss Agnes Nicholls, on the Friday. The Chairman of the Board, Sir William Cobbett, presided throughout. The Bazaar was held in the Out-Patients' Department, transformed and made gay with coloured streamers and balloons. There were fourteen stalls. The nurses had proved themselves adept not only at the creation of dainty garments, jumpers, frocks and hats, but also at jam-making, and their pots of home-made preserves were deservedly popular. There were stalls of china, basket work, hardware and dolls. The medical students showed much ingenuity in providing amusing sideshows in a tent on the lawn and their part of the Bazaar was well patronised. A sum of £4,500 was raised.

Early in 1923 Miss Sparshott was returned top of the poll at the recent election of the Council of the College of Nursing. The Board congratulated her but there was a difficulty. Sir Arthur Stanley asked permission for her to attend. Meetings were held on three Tuesdays and one Friday each month. This called for very careful consideration as to whether the Matron could be spared for so many days from Manchester, even though her attendance at the Council meetings had advantages for the Infirmary. In the end it was cautiously agreed to give her the necessary permission for six months. The hospital did not fall down and subsequently permission was extended annually.

Miss Sparshott, in 1923, reported that, owing to the difficulty in obtaining probationer nurses and to the number of sick and absent members of the staff, she was unable to give facilities for the remainder to take their annual holiday unless the Board of Management could assist by temporarily reducing the number of beds. The matter was referred to the House Committee and the Medical Board. Permission was refused.

The Royal Insurance Company notified the Board, in 1923, that the fire insurance of the building would not be affected in consequence of the installation of wireless in the hospital.

The Medical Board minutes for 1924 analyse the results of the final examination for nurses during the last five years:

	Passed	Failed
1919	37	3
1920	50	1
1921	51	2
1922	37	1
1923	29	1
	204	**8**

This was regarded as highly satisfactory but the housing of nurses was still a cause for much anxiety. During the past 10 years, up to 1924, twenty-five nurses had to be lodged, two and even three in a room, in a couple of small houses adjoining the hospital. There was concern too to establish a Preliminary Training School in which fifteen accepted probationers would undergo two months of preparation as an introduction to the duties which they would be called upon to perform immediately they embarked upon their training in the wards. The importance of this preliminary training could not be overstated.

There were 220 nurses in 1924. The reduction of working hours would mean the engagement of 72 additional nurses.

The first of a series of American tea-parties in connection with the College of Nursing was held in 1924.

A new qualifying examination for nurses began in 1925. Up to now nurses had qualified by passing examinations at the hospitals where they had trained, but unfortunately standards varied considerably. The new State examination had now to be passed before a nurse could receive her certificate. The General Nursing Council asked permission for this examination to be held at the Infirmary periodically and this was readily given.

The need for a new Nurses' Home was well shown by the following figures which were well advertised. Manchester, so accustomed to lead in all good works, was in the unenviable position of having to overwork its nurses:

Hospital	Hours of work	
	Day	Night
Aberdeen	52	52
Sheffield	56	64
Newcastle	60	73
Manchester	63	73

Appeals had now been issued for the necessary money. At first the cost of the new Home was £100,000, but by 1925 this had risen to £150,000 − £100,000 for the building and £50,000 for furniture and equipment. But money was slow in coming in. By January 1927, £57,200 had been subscribed, mostly by big business houses. This was delaying the laying of the foundation stone, but in due course Her Royal Highness Princess Mary, Viscountess Lascelles, performed the ceremony on May 14, 1927. It was laid many yards from its final resting-place. The Chairman reminded her that the King was a patron and that in 1909 King Edward VII and Queen Alexandra opened the present building. At that time it was thought there was ample accommodation for many years to come. Conditions had changed and in order to diminish the present working hours of the nurses to 56 hours a week it was necessary to add no fewer than 157 nurses and domestic servants to the staff. In addition, accommodation had to be found for 82 nurses and masseurs who who were temporarily lodged outside the Infirmary. As an encouragement to donors, rooms would be named after anyone who gave £500 or more.

While this was taking place Miss Sparshott's salary had been increased by £50, and she had had a serious operation which kept her off duty for three months.

The Board was asked in 1927 to support an application to the Privy Council for the granting of a Royal Charter to the College of Nursing. The Chairman was authorised to sign on behalf of the Board. The application succeeded.

It is interesting to find that Platt Hall was offered to the Board for the accommodation of their nursing staff. There were difficulties and the offer was regretfully declined. But three things were done to help the nurses and their training. A second-hand microscope was bought at a cost of £7 10s., alterations were made to their dining-hall at considerable expense and badges were awarded to nurses trained at the Infirmary. The year 1927 saw the retirement of Sister Lees after 39 years' service, and next year Sister Naden also after 39 years. We met her in uniform in 1902 in the operating theatre at the Old Infirmary (Figure 6).

The Medical Board now took a hand in progress by suggesting the formation of a small nursing sub-committee to consist of representatives of the Board of Management and the Medical Board. The Board at once agreed and each nominated representatives. It seems hard to believe that there had been no nursing committee until 1929. Arising out of this the Annual Report in future had a special section on the Nursing Service.

The Board decided to award an annual prize of £40 to the Nurse obtaining most marks in the final examination. The money had to be used towards some further course of training. A minimum of 75 per cent had to be paid direct to the teaching authority concerned. If the prize was not accepted it lapsed.

There was a reunion of Infirmary and Territorial Army Nursing Service Nurses in 1928. The Denton Prize Band were invited for a fee of £15.

Probationers' salaries were increased. First year probationers would receive £20, second year £25 and third year £30.

It was decided to install a fire alarm in the new Nurses' Home with three call switches on each of the five floors (15 altogether) at a cost of £118 3s.

A scheme for pensions for hospital officers and nurses was considered. The Secretary was asked to collect statistics from hospitals

in London and Norwich and provide details of the existing scheme
at the Infirmary and the amount paid annually in pensions. When
the figures were produced to the Infirmary Committee they were
referred to the Finance Committee, who took more than a year to
produce a scheme with the very active help of an Actuary.

November 27, 1928
The scheme took the form of superannuation and can be summarised
as follows:
(a) Future entrants into the service of the Infirmary after January 1,
1929, will be admitted to the Federated Superannuation Scheme of
Pensions for Nurses of which the principal provisions are set out in
Section A; and (b) Present members of the staff as at January 1, 1929,
will be treated as follows: 'Nurses, Sisters and Matrons who are at
present guaranteed a pension of £78 will be included in the Internal
Scheme as set out in Section B. Alternatively, and on request of the
member, the Federated Scheme may be applied in individual cases.'

(a) Future Entrants after January 1, 1929
Federated Scheme. The Federated Superannuation Scheme of Pensions
for Nurses will apply to all entrants into the service of the Infirmary
after January 1, 1929, as follows: Matrons, Sisters and Nurses – compulsory; Probationers (after one year's training) – optional on the part of
Infirmary during training, compulsory on appointment as a Nurse;
Probationers (first year) – ineligible.
Contributions. The annual contribution in each case is 15 per cent of
the total salary and emoluments apportioned as follows: Infirmary 10
per cent; Nurse 5 per cent. The value of the emoluments is reckoned
according to the scale set out in the Federated Scheme.
Benefits. The benefits take the form of an insurance policy of which
the member has some choice.
Migrations. Nurses migrating within the hospital service will take the
benefit of both contributions.
Withdrawals from the Hospital Service. A Nurse admitted to the
Scheme as a Probationer leaving the nursing service altogether will take
the benefit of both contributions, unless her withdrawal occurs within
five years of the completion of her training. In the latter case she will
take the benefit of her own contributions only. A nurse admitted to the
Scheme as a fully trained Nurse, leaving the nursing service altogether
will take both contributions, unless her withdrawal occurs within five
years of her admission to the Scheme. In the latter case she will take the
benefit of her own contributions only.
Death Benefits. If an employee dies after admission to the Scheme, the
proceeds of the policy will be paid to such member's legal representative.

(b) Existing Staff as at January 1, 1929

Nurses, Sisters and Matrons would be covered by an Internal Scheme under which no contributions will be paid by individual employees. But members of the Nursing Staff may elect at the outset to enter the Federated Scheme instead of the Internal Fund.

The Internal Scheme consists of the setting aside by the Infirmary of a certain sum of money to be accumulated at compound interest to provide a fund out of which annuities may be purchased on the retirement of members of the Scheme.

Pensions will be granted on retirement at pension age or earlier through ill health.

Contributions credited could be allowed under *Migration Benefit, Withdrawal from the Hospital Service* and *Death Benefits* as under Section (a).

The Actuary added an important Summary:

As regards those members of the staff who are not covered by the Federated Scheme, it will be observed that the Internal Scheme allows the Committee the most complete freedom of action. No trust is set up and no definite promises are made. The Infirmary is therefore not committed to any fixed rate of contribution. But I do urge the members to bear in mind the consideration that whereas the younger members of the staff are now provided with a generous means of building up pensions for their old age, present older members had no such opportunities in the past, and have now too short a period of future service in which to reap the benefits of the new scheme. Equity demands that the old servant should not be less generously treated than the new. The more so in view of the fact that the absence of provision for future pensions results not from any fault of the employee but rather from a lack of foresight, or a putting off of a responsibility on the part of the employer.

The Board accepted the Scheme.

Miss Sparshott resigned in March 1929. In the section that follows she is remembered by her nurses and those she worked with.

(e) Miss Sparshott remembered

My nursing experience in 1914 would shock the modern nurse. Who now-a-days would spend hours cleaning brasses and taps in bathrooms and dusting wards? It's 'not done' now. Besides, you could not smoke or entertain housemen except on the Q.T. As for being late on days out! Well that meant a visit to Miss Sparshott and a real telling off. And holidays were given to suit the hospital and not the nurse.

But you have pressed me to recall my nursing days. We wore gloves to try and keep our hands nice because of metal polish. I remember my feelings on my first ward, a male medical, my first introduction to men in shirts not pyjamas and having to make their beds. Within my first week we had a death from hæmorrhage and the young nurse ran to call Sister, while I did what I could. Old Sister Reid came sailing down the ward, calm and so gentle. You felt she knew her job and though the poor man died yet she was calm all through and afterwards called us into the linen room and said, 'Remember – never panic, never run, but come quietly and quickly. The only time you run is for fire.' I learnt a lot from her for she was a real martinet but taught well and you never forgot what she had said.

Nursing training in 1914 was very different from what it is today. The probationer went straight on to the wards. There was no preliminary training school for six months. The nurse studied and attended lectures in off-duty time. She came on duty at 7 a.m. having had breakfast, to do bedmaking, dusting and preparing trollies for treatment or for the surgeon. Lavatories and bathrooms had to be cleaned and the brasses polished. The ward maid only polished the floors and scrubbed the kitchen and corridor. Nurses had to turn out patients' lockers weekly, do the flowers, take meals to the patients and wash the sick ones. Probationers learnt to do bed-bathing and different treatments and how to give medicines and take temperatures.

Duty time was 7 a.m. to 8 p.m. with two hours off either in the afternoon or evening and you left the ward for half an hour for a midday meal either at 12-30 or 1-30 according to off-duty time. If off duty from 2-30 to 4-30 you went to the second dinner and had your tea before returning to the ward. If off duty from 6 p.m. to 10 p.m. you missed tea and had to wait for supper at 8-30 or get it with friends. The day staff had to have all beds made and patients washed before the night staff came on at 8 p.m.

There was a rest day once a month but this was apt to be missed if a war convoy was being admitted. The pro. got two weeks' holiday a year at a time to suit the Matron. You had to wear black stockings and low-heeled shoes. If you were caught smoking or entertaining a house-man you were sent to Matron and got into trouble.

The night nurse came on duty at 8 p.m. and worked to 8 a.m. There was one nurse to each ward with a junior nurse as 'runner' between two wards to help with heavy cases. The first job of the night nurse, after receiving the report, was to see that all patients were comfortably settled, then lower the lights and do night duty treatment, medicines, etc. In my time the night nurse took her night meal in the ward kitchen if and when she could leave the ward for half an hour in the care of the runner. Sometimes on an admission night she might only manage a cup of tea until going off duty to a meal at 9 a.m. The night nurse was responsible for washing all poorly patients and making their beds before the day staff arrived at 7 a.m. This often meant early washing if you had many serious cases but if you were caught doing this before 6 a.m. the Night Sister reported you. The Sister was on duty from 8 a.m. to 1 p.m. She was then off for two hours and back again for the evening. On alternate days she went off at 5 p.m. In her absence the staff nurse was in charge. Sisters had alternate weekends off duty. When Physicians or Surgeons did a ward round with Sister or Staff Nurse there had to be strict silence.

Theatre work was very heavy. The Sister came on at 8 a.m., the nurse at 7 a.m. She had to polish taps and sterilizers, get the instruments ready and help to get the drums sterilized. The theatre maid washed the floors and corridors. A nurse had to be ready scrubbed-up during operations to fetch and carry for the Sister and Surgeon or to assist in any way. You had to have a pass when you went out and the porter checked you when you came in. If late you had to go to Matron's office next morning and be told off. During the war when convoys came in day and night a nurse could be called from off-duty time or in the night. I lost many a half day because of this.

Miss Sparshott was so stiff and on her dignity that I never felt at home with her even when I was a staff nurse. She was so stern. She would run her finger along the radiators looking for dust and woe betide the nurse who failed to keep the electric light shades clean. Even the quilts had to be pocketed evenly and I was called up more than once to remake one. If you met her on the corridor you had to have a reason for being there and not on your ward and woe betide if you were hurrying. No excuse was accepted even though you had been sent to find a doctor. I ran right into her once when I was hurrying! I never got over my awe of her, but we adored Sister Smith, the Assistant Matron, and would do anything for her. To be sent to *her* in disgrace was a far greater punishment for she looked so sorry you had done anything wrong. I think Miss Sparshott tried to be fair but the work and the patients came first. Your own wants took second place. You might go with your Sister's permission to ask for a day off. She would refuse on the grounds that if your ward didn't want you, another ward did. The result was we didn't ask, we took what was given.

I wouldn't be a nurse today. I'd rather do the old hard work, for you felt so rewarded when you saw the result of your work. Whereas today I'm sure the senior nurses must get exasperated with girls who don't seem to take their work seriously.

Preparation. Like all little girls, my dolls played a part in my young life. From the age of 7 years I would imagine as I went out on an errand for mother, that I collected wounded and brought them home to nurse. I was very brave for I rode an imaginary horse. My father was interested in the St. John and Red Cross Societies, eventually winning the 25 years' Silver Medal on which was the engraving of the head of Florence Nightingale. My father would practise bandaging and pressure points on me, two things which helped me later in nursing.

The 1914 war increased my interest. I used to pass the M.R.I. on my way to work in an office in town, and see the wounded soldiers looking out of the front windows of the new Physiotherapy Department, thinking one day I will nurse in there. Little did I think that I should have to wait seven years, for no one was admitted until 21 years of age. In those days we could leave school in our 14th year, but before I finally left I won a scholarship for a short term of Domestic Science. Would I train for a teacher of Domestic Science? – No, I wanted to be a nurse.

It was now necessary to take a job of some kind and bring some money into the home. Was I to be a shop assistant or work in an office? The office was chosen and the training in office routine helped later in administrative posts. I well remember my first interview with my prospective employer. He said, 'So you are to be our new telephone girl.' 'Only until I can go to the Manchester Royal Infirmary,' I replied. The next seven years were spent in this office. I attended evening classes, where in addition to the subjects needed for the office I took other subjects which I thought would be useful in nursing. There was no one to guide us in those days, but, as Miss Sparshott pointed out to me at my interview, I had pulled myself up to secondary standard, without which she could not have taken me.

When the time came for me to give my notice to my employer, I told him that I was going to nurse at the M.R.I. He said that he thought that I had got the nonsense out of my mind. He predicted that I would stay three months, and said I could go back to my job with them. Some three years later I did return to see them and show my certificates and they followed my nursing career until the 2nd world war.

My first interview. With awe I stood outside the door of Matron's office at the end of the Medical corridor, and, bidden to enter, I saw behind the desk a trim small figure in a black dress and snowy lace cap and collar. After greetings and an invitation to sit down, she said suddenly, in her quick way, 'I see you sew.' Startled I wondered how she knew? She smiled, and as I looked at my fingers with the telltale needle pricks, I explained how I had been making moccasins for Christmas presents. From that moment my awe for Miss Sparshott's powers of observation never left me. On perusing the written information before her, she said 'You seem to be the right type of person, and your evening classes have brought you up to the standard required, and I see that you want to be a medical missionary, but there is one thing, I do not usually take girls from their own town, because you see there will be bright days and dark days and on dark days you might run home.' I assured her that I would be sent back. I was interested to learn that I was just half an inch taller than the required height, which was 5 foot 1.

Kind thought. Word came that I had been accepted for January 15, 1923, on which day I would be 22 years old. (21 was the minimum age for admission.) Matron suggested I had this birthday at home and start on the next day, which I thought was very kind.

Uniform. The uniform, which I was always proud to wear, had a shaped and lined bodice with puffed sleeves, a detachable part from the elbow, a very wide skirt with a 2 inch hem and three 1 inch tucks. Matron was very particular about this uniform, it had to be 8 inches from the ground and the apron hem 1 inch shorter. The aprons were made from very substantial material. Two sisters had a linen shop in the row of shops past Nelson Street. To these we took our material to be made up. They had broad waist bands with two buttons and button-holes. There was to be no belt added. Our stockings were black wool or cashmere, and were a great trial to nurses who wanted to wear silk. Shoes were black with cuban heels, and rubbers on the heels for, said matron, 'no noise was to be made when walking down a ward', and oh dear! if our shoes started to squeak.

Lectures. Matron gave us our first six lectures, and by that time she had weighed us up. From these lectures I have always remembered the one on the reverent laying out of the dead. Later we had Sister Abram as our sister tutor.

Deportment. Meeting Miss Sparshott on the corridor one day, she sharply remarked, 'Nurse you are walking like a barrel', then swiftly passed on.

Discipline. Hair was worn long, and we mostly had a bun. However short hair was becoming the fashion and two of our group had their hair cut, but wore a switch on duty. Alas one day it fell off in the ward, and matron showed her disapproval in no uncertain way. V.A.D. caps were issued to the offenders, or rather one cap which required washing and starching daily as punishment. It was about the time of our finals, but there were no strings for these two, and on our group photograph there they sit in our midst with V.A.D. caps. How times have changed! Make-up was also frowned upon, as one nurse found as she was about to leave the M.R.I. off duty. She was sent back to remove it, and yet, was it the Christmas spirit that a few weeks before my finals, at Roby Street Matron caught me on top of a ladder putting up decorations, a rather dishevelled nurse; on my cheek a black patch stuck on by one of the male patients. Was it the Christmas spirit that made her remark 'At last they have brought you out.' Much to my confusion. We had one fancy-dress dance at Christmas, but we had been so long in uniform that we felt awkward in evening or fancy dress, and yet they were fun.

Matron must have had a hard time to keep watch that no houseman slipped in in fancy dress, for nurses and housemen were not to mix.

Church. Each time I go to the re-union service, I look up to the organ loft and in my memory I see Miss Sparshott playing the hymns and looking down at her nurses, and woe betide if one fell asleep. Yet after a night on duty and a good dinner – oh dear!

Training for Service. Never shall I forget the rebuke I got when I had become dissatisfied with my continual changing of wards. For a period I was to start at S.1. on their accident receiving day, leave there at 10 a.m. next day and proceed to S.2. and so to each unit, then back to S.1. and so start the circle again. It seemed to me that any missing article was lost on the day I was on the ward, or maybe some patient's toe nails had been missed. Night duty was similar. Every two nights on the next ward where someone had a night off. 'Why does matron not give you a settled ward?' asked some of my fellow nurses. That 'why not?' grew bigger in my mind every day. Until Matron stopped me on the corridor to ask why I looked so miserable. I said that I was wondering why I had not a settled ward like other nurses. 'You want to be a missionary nurse?' 'Yes,' I replied. 'Well, I'm training you for one, now get on with your work.' I was very grateful for this training when I did arrive in the Middle East.

The Royal College of Nursing. I recall how very enthusiastic Miss Sparshott was for the College of Nursing as it was then known. She encouraged us to join at the end of our training, which I did in 1926, and I have been a full member until last year when I was put on the associate members' list. What a joy it would have been for her to know that the Royal College has been of so much service to so many, and reached its Jubilee.

An introduction to nursing, 1923

January 16, 1923. I, along with three other young ladies, arrived at the Manchester Royal Infirmary, and was conducted to the old Nurses' Home. Previously we had been measured and provided with our striped mauve and white dress and aprons, which we had paid for ourselves, only to be given the same uniform some three months later if we were finally accepted. We were shown to our bedrooms, told to put on this uniform and await the Home Sister. This we did, but how was the cap, which lay flat open, to be made into the shape required? Sister came, took a tooth brush and damped the starch round the tapes so allowing the cap to be gathered, then with our hair combed straight back and into a bun, the cap was perched on the top and secured with two pins, and one looked into the mirror to see oneself looking very starched, but very proud.

Next day. Called at 6 a.m. Breakfast 6-30 a.m. Then ward allocation. I found that I was to go to S.3.F. I was taken in hand by a probationer six months my senior, a very kind young lady, who regretfully had to give up nursing because of heart trouble. We found ourselves in a stream of nurses all going to their wards. There was no preliminary training school.

First day on the ward. On arrival at S.3.F. I was instructed to take off the half sleeves and cuffs and leave them in the Linen Room. Then the ward. It seemed tremendous to me as I walked down to the far end to start bed making. A senior nurse took me to the right side of beds and soon I was shown how to fold the bedclothes over two chairs at the foot of the bed, the mystery of a draw sheet, and the remaking of the bed, and so on down the ward, each bed being pulled away from the wall. The speed of the procedure amazed me, and later I realised how exasperating must have been the first attempts at bed-making on a busy ward. I was shown a mysterious brush called 'Long Tom', with which the walls were brushed once a week. Then the very wide floor brush. The procedure was to sweep behind the beds in one quick walk from the door to the fireplace. Then dust and put back the beds making sure that the castors at the foot of the bed were turned in. Back for the brush to sweep the dust into the middle of the ward. Now under the furniture in the centre of the ward using straight strokes backwards and forwards. Now came the race, each nurse placing her brush before her walked quickly up and down the space between the bed ends and the centre furniture. So the ward was swept. Next the centre furniture was dusted, and one was ready for the arrival of Sister, or should have been. Alas, my side was far from finished.

Sister Lees. Sister sat down at the table in the centre of the ward to take the night nurse's report and give instructions for the day. Only then did we know the time of our two hours off duty. This 'not knowing' was a trial we had to endure throughout our training. Sister Lees was an elderly sister, who wore her dress down to the floor. She appeared formidable to me that day, but I can remember her smile and quick speech and silvery chuckle on occasions, to this day.

The day continued. Next we went off in turn for half an hour for a snack, and to make our own beds and change aprons. The day that followed was a nightmare of people calling 'Nurse do this' or that, or fetch this or that, and one must have been a nuisance on this Theatre day on S.3.F. because in those days Sister or Staff nurse assisted in the Theatre with one ward probationer, and so on this day the ward was more depleted of staff than ever. I was sent round to collect an egg off each person able to have one beaten into their morning milk. I was introduced to the sluice work where piles of sheets were sluiced before

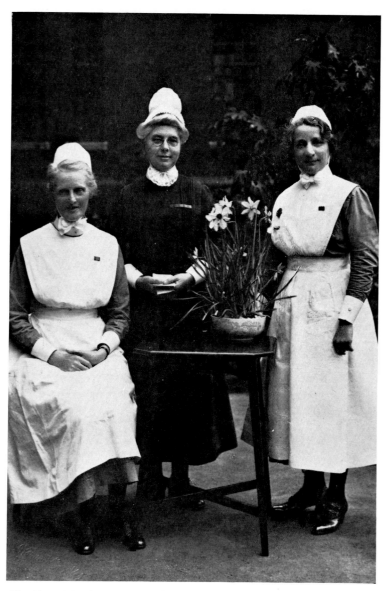

10 Sister Mundy, Miss Sparshott and Sister Overstall

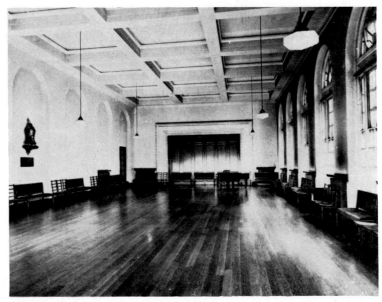

11 The Great Hall as it was in 1932 and is now

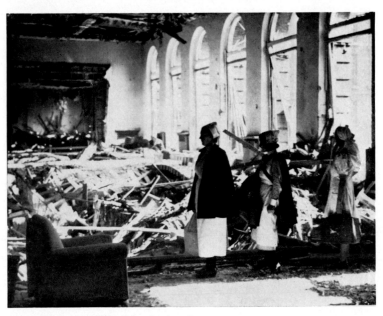

12 The Great Hall after the bomb

being sent to the laundry, and the dressing trolley was cleaned. This was one of the places Matron would visit on her morning round. All the time the patients were being prepared for the Theatre and whisked away on a trolley, to be brought back and slid on to specially prepared beds.

Two amusing incidents. Two distinct incidents stand out in my memory (remember I had not been on a ward before):

(1) I was instructed to 'Watch that patient does not pull out her tubes.' I gazed at the tubes from a drip which disappeared under the bed clothes and wondered where they went to.

(2) A patient returned from the theatre with an airway. I was told to watch her as often the patients were restless on returning to consciousness after ether. Timidly I went to the Linen room and asked if it was all right for the patient to be vomiting through this airway? 'Pull it out.' Then remembering it was my first day someone came to the rescue, and so I saw a complete airway. How good it must be today to have a training school, and not need to be made to feel useless.

Afternoon and evening. The patients' dinner trolley came, and we put on our sleeves and cuffs, and tried to remember which dinner belonged to which patient. Then our dinner time came and we walked again to the Nurses' dining room with the clatter of nurses and plates. Some of us then had our two hours off, which I spent lying on my bed with shoes off until tea-time. Back to the ward and another round of bed making, patients' suppers, and at 8 p.m. all patients settled and lights out, except for the shaded light above the Sister's table. The night nurses arrived and we day ones went to supper and to our rooms. A bath and 10 p.m. Home Sister's knock and to tell us lights out. I went to bed stiff and tired and soon slept, only to be called next morning with the familiar sound of 'six o'clock nurse', and another day began and I wondered if the stiffness would allow me to work. But another round of bed-making, etc. soon made me fit again. How much easier it is for all concerned to have the present preliminary training school. We had the first Sister Tutor in Sister Abram.

Weekly routine. In addition to the daily work of the ward, each week certain things had to be done on certain days, i.e., electric shades over beds to be cleaned, and glass doors for which one tried to get some methylated spirit on one's cloth to speed up the job. There were the lockers and linen rooms to be cleaned.

Aspidistras. In the centre of the ward was a large table with many plants in fancy plant bowls. Once a week these were taken on the tea trolley to the bathroom. The plants were put into the bath, water up to the brims, and left while other work was done. Then the fancy bowls

H

were washed with soap and water as were all the leaves, then all were returned to the ward, in time to release the trolley for ward teas.

Impossible? 'What have you been doing Nurse? Look at the time.' 'But I can't do all that before tea' brought the answer, 'You will', and I did.

Eggs. There were 24 eggs collected from the patients, these were to be beaten up for Egg Flip at 10 a.m. The 24 mugs were on the trolley. While I was making a great clatter beating these, Sister Lees came into the kitchen. Taking a mug and fork she showed me a quieter and more efficient way to get air into it.

'No noise please'. All was quiet, the Senior Doctor with many students was explaining a case to them and I was all ears behind the screen. Having finished the bed bath I picked up the bowl and silently made my way to the sluice; alas, I slipped and oh! the noise as I sat in the bowl; oh! the mess and the embarrassment as the students came to pick me up. Another occasion was at night. A very special patient was in a medical side ward. Instructions were 'to be kept very quiet'. All went well until the fire had to be made up, and in my nervousness I dropped the whole shovel of coal in the hearth.

Coal fires. The night runner had to make up the ward fires twice during the night and the nurse on M.2. unit had also the septic block (now the Neuro-Surgical), 13 fires in all.

Kindness. I would pay tribute to my first Staff Nurse, Nurse Chubb, who taught me with kindness and understanding, including my first introduction to death and the last offices. Even so it took courage to re-enter that silent room and empty the locker.

Night duty. It was in the quiet when alone one walked down the ward, speaking a comforting word, or re-arranging a pillow, etc., that one felt not alone but that a Divine Presence was with one.

(f) Time-tables and Ward Staff

Lectures.

1st Year. Matron's lectures. Bed making. Care of the ward. A course of lectures on hygiene given by the Theatre Sister, who was also in charge of the Maids' home. Anatomy lectures (12) given by a Surgeon. The Sister Tutor gave a revision after each lecture. If you failed the Anatomy examination you had to leave. The Preliminary State examination was taken at the end of the first year. If failed twice you were required to leave.

2nd Year. Medical lectures given by a Physician. Sister Tutor gave revision classes.

3rd Year. Special lectures. As far as I can remember there were 4 Gynæcology; 4 Ophthalmic; 2 Radiology; 2 Anæsthetic; 2 Physiotherapy. The Sister Tutor gave revision classes. At the end of the third year, Hospital Finals, State Finals. The P.T.S. only came into being in 1931 as far as I can recollect.

Ward Staff

Surgical Wards. Double lobby wards: 1 Sister, 2 staff nurses, 3 Probationers on day duty. 2 Probationers on night duty, 1 Probationer (runner) on a unit. Single lobby wards: 1 Sister, 1 Staff nurse, 2 Probationers on day duty. 1 Probationer 3rd year on night duty, 1 Probationer (runner) from the double lobby ward at certain times.

Medical Wards. As single lobby wards.

Theatres. 1 Staff nurse and 1 Probationer.

Accident Room. 1 Sister, 1 Staff nurse, 2 Probationers; Sister from Out Patients relieved Sister off duty.

Out Patients' Department. 1 Sister, 2 Staff nurses, 4 Probationers.

Night Staff. Surgical side: 1 Night Sister, 1 Staff nurse, 1 Theatre Staff nurse, 1 3rd year Probationer on the Accident Room. Medical side: 1 Night Sister, 1 Night Staff nurse.

Off Duty

Sisters. 1-30 – 4-30 p.m., or off duty 4-30 p.m.

Staff nurses. The same.

Probationers. 9-30 a.m. – 12-30 p.m., 1-30 – 4-30 p.m., lunch and teatime and sometimes a lecture during this period; or 4-30 – 6-30 p.m., usually a lecture. Very occasionally an evening off, 6-30 p.m. All lectures were taken during 'off duty'. All day staff had one half day a month, one day off a month, and alternate Sundays, half a day.

Night staff. Two nights off a month for all, including the Night Sister.

Duty Times

Sisters, on duty 8 a.m. Took reports from the night nurse, made out the diet sheet for the kitchen, bulletin for Nelson Street lodge, orders for the various departments, lists of work for the nurses, and did a round of the patients. Doctors' rounds 9 a.m.

Staff nurses, on duty 7 a.m. Made half the ward beds with the junior probationer, took all patients' temperatures at the same time as making the beds, did the flowers. Prepared for dressings and treatments.
9 a.m. Went for coffee, and made her own bed.
9-30. Treatments for the patients. Before going for coffee she prepared patients for the Theatre.

Probationers on duty 7 a.m. Collected the used tea leaves from the kitchen, pulled out one side of beds and furniture, one probationer made beds with the Staff nurse and one with the Night nurse. Swept behind the beds and dusted them and put them back. She then scattered the tea leaves and swept the rest of the floor. This had to be completed before Sister appeared at 8 a.m.

8 a.m. One probationer to clean the bathroom, and one the sluice. They did all the cleaning but for the floors and brasses.

9 a.m. Patients' drinks, patients' backs, and tidy the beds. Sweep the floors again but without the tea leaves.

9 – 9-30 or 9-30 – 10. Coffee. Make her own bed and tidy her room. Change her apron. Do the ward messages. On her return, if she was lucky she might be allowed to help with dressings or treatments, or she may be the Theatre-ward probationer for the day, otherwise she would do the extra work.

12. Patients' dinners.

12-45 – 1-15. Go to lunch, or 1-30 go to lunch and off duty until 4-30. After the patients had lunch, tidy beds and sweep the floor. During the afternoon, extra work.

4 p.m. Patients' teas. Wash the patients' hands and face, make the beds and attend to patients' backs. Sweep the wards.

6-30 p.m. Patients' drinks. Help with the evening treatments, tidy the bathroom and sluice.
Bed-pan rounds were done at 9 a.m. and 12-30, after tea, and again during the evening. The ward was closed during the bed-pan rounds.

Extra work. Monday. The linen room shelves were scrubbed. Other days. Sweep the ward walls, this took two afternoons. Wash the electric light shades, polish all the furniture, clean the ward radiators, clear out the clothes room. All bandages were washed and ironed by the nurses.

Night staff on duty 9 p.m. – 8-15 a.m. They were responsible for preparing the soiled linen for the Sister or Staff nurse to count in the morning. Ward mending. The care of the patients was their chief concern.

(g) Three of My Own Memories

Sister Simpson
There was an earlier Sister Simpson who had been something of a legend at the Old Infirmary. My Sister Simpson used to be night sister on the medical corridor and had the reputation of being difficult. I encountered her on my first night as house physician and

she sailed into the attack. I had prescribed digitalis for a patient and she did not approve. Luckily, she was so obviously wrong that I stood my ground and won the battle. I never had any more trouble with her and, as I got to know her, I appreciated her very many good qualities.

I knew her best three years later when I became R.M.O., and was frequently astonished at how much local colour she knew. I remember one night going to her office (the room now occupied by the Professor of Medicine). I wanted to see a patient on M.3F. and knew she would like to come with me. She said that it was awkward because Mr. ... was gossiping with the night nurse in the ward kitchen. After a pause she seized the telephone and asked for the ward. When the nurse replied she enquired if the R.M.O. had been. The answer, of course was 'No'. She then said that I was coming to see the patient in a minute or two and would she detain me until she came along. We waited a minute and then went upstairs together. We passed Mr. ... coming down all smiles. So too were we a moment later.

There was another occasion when she said, 'Do you want to see something that will interest you?' Always game, I said I did. She took me to the junction of the Nelson Street and Oxford Road corridors. It was nearly 11 p.m. 'Now,' she said, 'Any minute Nurse Jones will come in from Nelson Street.' Nurse Maud Jones was the staff nurse at that time; very efficient, very pleasant and quite adept at tennis. Within a minute we saw her coming – she passed us with a ravishing smile and a cheery 'Good night!' 'Now,' said Sister Simpson, 'Mr. Morris will come in from Oxford Road.' Again she was right. He too approached us grinning and turned left for the Accident Room, for he was the Assistant R.S.O. She made no comment. But it was the first I knew of an impending engagement that grew into a happy marriage. Little did either of them know why we were standing there.

There was another amusing incident connected with matrimony. It was a strict, unwritten rule that the R.M.O. and R.S.O. should not be married. Towards the end of my period of office it became clear that the R.S.O. had been secretly wed. Phone calls came to me asking for Mr. Scotson or his wife. When I protested that he had no wife I was put very clearly in the picture. Fearing that other people would get similar calls I thought I had better tackle him on the subject. He said that it was quite true and he wanted to let the cat out of the bag somehow. I undertook to do this at once.

Sister Whitfield on M.1F. was just the right person for that sort of job. So I told her the story and asked her to spread the news in the Nurses' Home – but nothing happened. After three days the R.S.O. asked me to try again. This time I went to Sister Simpson and told her the story, adding details about my first abortive attempt to spread the news. It was clear that Jessie hadn't believed me and this amused Sister Simpson vastly. She did the job splendidly.

Have you ever caught a night sister fast asleep on duty? I did once. I curbed very strongly the desire to waken her, preferring to ring her up from a nearby phone. 'Oh, are you there, Sister! Can we go to M.2 to see a patient?' I gave her five minutes to recover and all was well and smiling when I returned. She was a good sort and very capable.

The Lady Superintendent

My first and last encounters as R.M.O. with Miss Sparshott, the Matron, were both memorable. She was a formidable person dressed in black, frilly, straightlaced blouse and skirt with a white lace cap perched on the top of her white hair (Figure 10). She was a strict disciplinarian, and there was an iron curtain between the nursing staff on one side and the residents on the other.

I took up my post in January 1927, a week or two before the total eclipse of the sun was due to take place visible in this country. The residents had arranged a chara party to Giggleswick Scar. The Sisters had also arranged to see the eclipse from the same place. Two completely independent parties. The eclipse was due to be complete shortly after sunrise. It seemed a pity that both parties could not mix from the start. They were clearly going to mix on the Scar. I was asked by residents and sisters to call on Miss Sparshott and see what could be done about it, but hopes were at zero. I approached her with my tail very much between my legs and explained the point and what we would like. She breathed a great sigh of relief and said, 'Oh! I am so glad. I didn't like the idea of my girls being alone in such a crowd.' The word 'girl' was amusing for most of the sisters were very far from being chickens. She went straight ahead with arrangements. We had a buffet supper before leaving and the last thing we saw from our mixed charas was Miss Sparshott waving a white handkerchief on the steps of the main entrance. It remains to be said that the outing was completely successful and a lifelong memory, for we saw the eclipse to perfection, which was more than a lot of people did.

Our final encounter was on my last night. In order to organise effective Christmas processions by the residents I borrowed from the Matron of Barnes Hospital complete uniforms of a sister, two nurses and a ward maid. Certain conditions were imposed which were easy to carry out. One of them was that I should hand them over to the Home Sister when my appointment ended. So having warned Sister Overstall (Figure 10) and waited until it was dark I unpacked the uniforms, put the dresses over one arm, the caps in one hand and, with cap-strings dangling from the other, I entered the Nurses' Home and knocked on Sister Overstall's door. It opened immediately and I found myself facing the Matron. There was an embarrassed moment of silence and she said, 'I'd better not ask any questions,' and hurried past me.

She had quite a surprising and unexpected sense of humour when she permitted it to appear. On one Christmas morning one of the residents, Godfrey Jones, dressed as a flapper for the Christmas procession – wide-eyed, long pigtails, short skirts, he looked the part to perfection. He had dressed in my sitting-room, which was next to Miss Sparshott's suite, and was rather late. As he left my room she left her suite, and being properly scandalised at what she saw, she followed 'her' from the residency to M.3 linen room, where 'she' was awaiting the arrival of the procession. Miss Sparshott sailed in after him and said, 'My dear, your skirt is far too short.' Godfrey turned round and burst out laughing and the Matron disappeared. Before I could tell the story to the nursing hierarchy she had told them herself with much laughter.

Sister Farrow

Mention of Dr. Jones reminds me of another story. He was House Physician on M.2 and very well liked. One day he asked Sister Farrow to get the apparatus ready for exploring an empyema and named the time. Through no fault of his own he turned up an hour late to be told that the R.M.O. had done the job. A test-tube of yellow purulent-looking material was produced. I never heard exactly what he said about me but it was quite something, until he was aware of twinkling eyes and suspicious grins. He then uncorked the tube and smelled it. It was full of soup.

Godfrey would never accept defeat without a struggle. Two days later he got his revenge. I had ordered two leeches out of sheer interest to be used on an hysterical patient. They came in a little chip box which also contained a wad of wool. On opening the box in the linen-room he saw only one. 'One had escaped!' In less time than it takes to tell the Nursing Staff, including Sister Farrow, were standing on the top of the drawers and on chairs holding their skirts tightly round their legs in a highly agitated manner. I always wished I had been there. After a few minutes Godfrey was unable to suppress laughter. He knew well that the other leech was hiding under the wool. Honours were even.

(h) 1929 and After

Board Meeting

The following letter was read from Miss M. E. Sparshott, C.B.E., R.R.C., resigning from the office of Lady Superintendent of Nurses.

> The Royal Infirmary,
> Manchester.
> March 25, 1929.

Dear Mr. Goldschmidt,

I shall have completed 21 years as Lady Superintendent of Nurses on October 1, 1929, and shall be glad if you and the Board will release me on that date.

I am naturally very sorry that I cannot see the New Home in working order, but it will be at least two years before it is ready, and the Matron who starts the new work will need at least two years to get the whole working well. By my resigning this year my successor will have ample opportunity of seeing how the nursing is done now, and be able to make her plans for the future.

It is needless for me to say how sad I feel at giving up my very happy sphere of work, but I shall be 60 next year, and a woman of over 60 is too old to continue this great work. I am writing at so early a date so that you will have ample time to find my successor.

> I am, yours sincerely,
> (Signed) *M. E. Sparshott.*

R. P. Goldschmidt, Esq.,
Chairman of the Board of Management,
Manchester Royal Infirmary.

On the Motion of the Chairman, Seconded by the Deputy-Chairman, it was *Resolved*: That the resignation of Miss M. E. Sparshott, C.B.E., R.R.C., Lady Superintendent of Nurses since 1907 be accepted with sincere regret. The Board desire to place on record their great appreciation of the valuable work performed by Miss Sparshott during her tenure of office. During the whole of this long period Miss Sparshott has fully deserved, and possessed, the absolute confidence of the Board, and has carried out her duties to their entire satisfaction. She has displayed administrative abilities of quite a remarkable order, coupled with a kindly tactful control of her subordinates, which has secured their loyal obedience, and inspired their affection and regard. The Board fully recognise that they are indebted to Miss Sparshott's conspicuous ability and untiring energy for the high position the Manchester Royal Infirmary occupies among the Nurse Training Schools of the country, and they feel that her retirement is a very serious loss to the Institution. Miss Sparshott's uniform kindness and courtesy and her sympathetic assistance in times of stress or difficulty will be long remembered by all who have been associated with her in the work of the Infirmary, and she will carry with her their most cordial wishes for her health and happiness.

Resolved: That a copy of the above Resolution be sent to Miss Sparshott and that a pension of £300 per annum be granted to Miss Sparshott in recognition of her eminent services to the Institution.

Miss Sparshott thanked the Board for the Resolution and the pension. At a later date the Board presented her with a clock and barometer.

The Medical Board desired to express their high appreciation of the long and faithful services of Miss M. E. Sparshott, 'who for 22 years has had charge of the Nursing Department of this hospital, and to pay a tribute to her energy and capability. They assure her that she will long be remembered for the excellent work she has performed and that she carries with her, to her well-earned leisure, the hearty appreciation and good wishes of those who have been associated with her in her professional life'.

It was decided to make a presentation to her and this took the form, at her own request, of 'a wireless apparatus' with a suitable inscription attached to it.

Miss Sparshott also resigned her post as principal matron of the Territorial Army Nursing Service for the Second Western General Hospital. Formed in 1908, with Miss Sparshott as the organising matron, it quickly enrolled its full compliment of sisters and nurses. During the war the sick and wounded dealt with by the Second Western General Hospital and its auxiliary hospitals was larger than any other general hospital in the country, a record in considerable measure due to the efficient administration of Miss Sparshott.

So much for local feeling. She was a national figure and *The Nursing Mirror and Midwives Journal* had this to say about her:

It is not only at her own hospital that Miss Sparshott's work has been of such outstanding merit. Her activities have extended to a wider sphere. She has always been ready to express an opinion forcibly and openly on any matter of importance to nurses. Fear of criticism has never held her silent. She has staunchly upheld the reputation of the provincial training schools and kept their affairs well to the fore. On the General Nursing Council on which body she has served from its inception in 1919, she has in fact, since the last election in 1927, been the sole representative of the provinces on the active list of matrons. She has proved a most energetic member of the Council especially on the Education and Examination Committee and, in spite of the fact that Manchester is a long way from London and of her onerous duties as Matron of a very large hospital, she has attended 69 Council meetings out of a total of 103.

There were still six months to pass before she departed. There was time for her to hold another bazaar in an attempt to collect £1,200 to ensure the provision in the new Home of a hall which would be a social and recreational centre for the nurses. It took place in May 1929 and she was very much the driving force behind it. Lord Derby performed the Opening Ceremony. It was immensely successful, £1,736 being raised.

She left on October 1 and there was very real regret and sadness at her departure even among those who had at times thought she was unduly strict. To do her job properly she had to be strict. There was little evidence that she had been unfair.

The new Nurses' Home was opened by the Lord Mayor on November 6, 1932, under the Chairmanship of the Chancellor of the University, the Earl of Crawford and Balcarres, P.C., K.T. Tribute was first paid to Mr. R. P. Goldschmidt, the Chairman of the Building Committee, for it was due to his foresight and courage that the scheme for building the Home was launched, backed by his patient and unostentatious work, that pushed the project through. There was 600 guests in the Great Hall which had been provided by past and present Nurses and Masseuses, who had contributed the sum of £10,653.

Miss Sparshott had returned to present the prizes and she received a very warm welcome. She said:

The M.R.I. has the reputation of being one of the best Nurse Training Schools in the country. During her training the Nurse has every opportunity of seeing the best work of physicians and surgeons and is taught the latest methods of nursing. She is coached throughout her career by a fully qualified Sister Tutor. Her health is always watched with the greatest care and arrangements are made for her to join the Federated Superannuation Scheme and so provide for her future. She enjoys many social advantages which will be increased by the additional staff which can now be accommodated in this magnificent new Home. M.R.I. Nurses are placed all over the world and are acting in all departments of nursing. Matrons of several hospitals in Britain, the late Matron-in-Chief of Lady Minto's Indian Nursing Association, the Matron-in-Chief of the Southern Rhodesian Nursing Service, the Matron of the Presidency General Hospital Calcutta, the Matron of the Somerset Hospital Capetown, and of several other hospitals overseas, all owe their training to the M.R.I. The work which demands the greatest self-sacrifice is that of the Missionary Nurse and we have at least fourteen in Africa, China and India. The Colonies and the United States of America also have a goodly number.

It was a triumphant meeting but alas there was one big snag. There was a deficiency of £67,000 on the Building Fund. The Home contained 400 rooms and housed 266 persons, including first, second and third-year probationers, staff nurses, sisters and assistant matrons. Each nurse had her own room. Eighty new nurses were added to the staff as a result of the new accommodation. Thus at last the whole nursing staff were gathered under one roof in York Place with opportunities of recreational and social life in off-duty periods which had hitherto been unavailable. The chief feature was its lofty, spacious Great Hall (Figure 11) which was given by the Nurses themselves and which bore a bronze tablet with the following inscription: 'In grateful recognition of the help and generosity of the nursing and massage staffs under the direction of Miss M. E. Sparshott, C.B.E., R.R.C., who contributed £10,653 to defray the cost of this hall.' The building had been so soundly constructed that it withstood the explosion inside it of a high calibre bomb during an air raid in World War II (Figure 12).

There is a note from one of her nurses which gives us a picture of Miss Sparshott in retirement:

Miss Sparshott had retired to her home in Penge, and on my furlough from the Middle East she invited me to speak at her church, and to stay the weekend with her friend and herself. What a friendly person she seemed now to me. Could it be my Matron who invited me to 'run and put your dressing gown on and come and drink your evening cup of milk before the fire?' Was she remembering her training days when the greatest pleasure was to take off the uniform and relax in a dressing gown maybe in a nurse friend's bedroom? Could it be my Matron placing a hot-water bottle in my bed, and bringing up my breakfast on a tray next morning? How pleased she was to show the gifts she had received on her retirement, and her garden. At the meeting at the church she introduced me as 'One of *my nurses* who was privileged to go to the Holy Land.' A place she had wanted to visit herself.

She died on October 9, 1940, two days before the Great Hall, for which she had done so much, was wrecked by the bomb which exploded within its walls. But the Hall has been restored to its former glory.

Index

Italic figures refer to illustrations